How to Dismantle the NHS in 10 Easy Steps

Youssef El-Gingihy

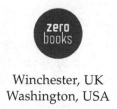

Winchester, UK
Washington, USA

First published by Zero Books, 2015
Zero Books is an imprint of John Hunt Publishing Ltd., Laurel House, Station Approach,
Alresford, Hants, SO24 9JH, UK
office1@jhpbooks.net
www.johnhuntpublishing.com
www.zero-books.net

For distributor details and how to order please visit the 'Ordering' section on our website.

ISBN: 978 1 78535 045 0
Library of Congress Control Number: 2015931661

A CIP catalogue record for this book is available from the British Library.

Design: Lee Nash

Printed and bound by CPI Group (UK) Ltd, Croydon, CR0 4YY, UK

We operate a distinctive and ethical publishing philosophy in all
areas of our business, from our global network of authors to
production and worldwide distribution.

CONTENTS

Dedicated to all those who have fought for the NHS and to a future NHS for all time.

I would like to thank those, who showed the way and illuminated my understanding of what has been happening to our NHS. It is only through their contribution that I have been able to write this book. All those years ago, they were lone voices. More people are now becoming aware of the marketisation and privatisation of the NHS and are determined to fight against vested interests to preserve it.

Introduction

I am a doctor. I work as a GP in London. Like most of you, I was born in a National Health Service hospital. I studied medicine and worked as a junior doctor in the NHS. I wrote this book because I fear that there will not be an NHS as our generation grows old and certainly not for our children. Yet the British public remains largely unawares of this and the media, with few exceptions, have failed in their duty to inform them. The remit of my book is charting how the NHS has been insidiously converted into a market-based healthcare system over the past 25 years. This process is accelerating under the Coalition government and the very existence of a National Health Service is in danger. This matters to all who use the NHS or are concerned by the privatisation of public services and the dismantling of equitable healthcare and welfare. The NHS—long the envy of the world—is being broken up into a universal insurance system based on the US model. Multinationals are opening the NHS oyster following on from the Health & Social Care Act 2012 and in preparation for the forthcoming Transatlantic Trade & Investment Partnership (TTIP EU-US trade agreement). This is about much more than the NHS; it is about turbo-charged neoliberalism—the ideological doctrine that encompasses privatisation, deregulation and shrinking the state.

We are on the eve of an epoch-defining general election in 2015. Put simply, this election is likely to define whether the NHS continues to exist as a cherished institution or whether it is gradually dismantled into a privatised, insurance-based system. The election, in the context of the financial crisis and austerity, would seem to be as significant as 1979. The issues at stake extend to the current neoliberal political and economic model and the kind of society we want to live in. It is likely to have huge ramifications for the direction Britain is heading in, at a time of

1

great change, turmoil and chaos across the world.

NHS politics is an area that can be dry and foreboding to the public. The concept of this book is to make it accessible and to communicate clearly what is happening to our NHS. I want to shine a light on the deliberate destruction of the nation's most sacred institution whilst the majority of the British public have been kept in the dark by a neoliberal agenda pursued by the main political parties and the media. I only became aware of what was happening in 2011 at the time that the Health & Social Care Bill was making its way through Parliament. Incredibly, they don't really teach you much at medical school or as a junior doctor about how the NHS works and the history of its evolution. Maybe they should—there's certainly enough time in five years of studying.

Healthcare affects us and our loved ones arguably more than anything else in our lives. It would be a tragedy if the NHS were to be dismantled by vested interests—to great detriment to all of us—without the British public even having a say in the matter. People often feel impotent in the face of powerful interests. Yet the NHS belongs to us and we are the only ones who can fight for and save it.

Lots of questions are being asked of the NHS by politicians, the media and the public, such as:

- Can the NHS survive the current crisis?
- Is the NHS affordable?
- Where will the money come from?
- Would we be better off with universal private insurance?
- I will try to answer them in this book. But what if these are the wrong questions diverting us from the real issues?

The National Health Service was created in 1948. It is one of the pillars of the welfare state. It was created as part of a planned economy to rebuild Britain after World War II. It is based on the principles of **universal, comprehensive, free healthcare** from cradle to grave with equity of care. It is part of our social fabric— 'a fundamental component of solidarity and equal citizenship'.[1]

The founder of the NHS, Aneurin Bevan, officially opened the first NHS hospital—Park Hospital in Manchester—on 5 July 1948. He met a 13-year-old girl with a liver condition by the name of Sylvia Diggory (née Beckingham), who became the first patient to be treated under the NHS. Ironically, the birthplace of the NHS, now renamed Trafford General, is one of many hospitals facing cuts and closures.[2]

Aneurin Bevan—a coal miner's son who fought hard against bitter opposition to establish the NHS—told her that it was a **'milestone in history—the most civilised step any country has ever taken'**. So, one day there was no such thing as the NHS and the next day it had come into existence. 1 April 2013—the day the Health & Social Care Act came into effect—represents the reversal of that process.

The Health & Social Care Act is virtually impenetrable, but the main thrust of it is: Primary Care Trusts and Strategic Health Authorities will be disbanded. In their place, Clinical Commissioning Groups (CCGs) will control about £60-80 billion of the NHS budget and commission local services. Commissioning will take place through competitive tendering of NHS contracts open to the voluntary and private sectors. **But these recent events are the final stages in a journey that started over 25 years ago...**

Although nobody has told you this, the NHS has been effectively abolished. The national in National Health Service has been removed. It is fast becoming more of a notional health service subject to the whims of commissioners, cuts and rationing.

Now that may seem like a strange thing to say, seeing as you can still go to your local GP or hospital and receive free healthcare. On the surface, nothing seems to have changed. But, as you read on, you will discover that everything has. It will take many years for this to become apparent. The NHS lives on as a logo, which has helped to keep the public in the dark.

Our story really starts in the 1980s with Margaret Thatcher. Speaking at the 60th anniversary of the NHS in 2008, Kenneth Clarke remarked that: 'In the late 1980s I would have said it is politically impossible to do what we are now doing'.[3]

Ken Clarke was talking about how the NHS has been gradually converted into a market-based healthcare system. After 30 years of neoliberalism, what was once impossible has become possible. Ken Clarke, of course, was there at the beginning. As Health Secretary under Thatcher, he got the ball rolling by introducing the internal market into the NHS in 1990.

Step One:
Create an Internal Market

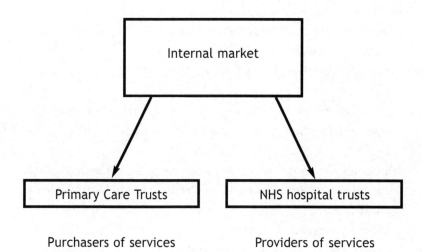

The 1980s saw the outsourcing of non-clinical hospital services like catering, cleaning and laundry. Under John Major, most NHS bodies were made into trusts. NHS hospital trusts—or providers—run by boards of governors and chief executives 'sold' their services to purchasers i.e. Primary Care Trusts. This became known as the purchaser-provider split. This means that hospitals have to compete against each other to get business. Except the NHS is not the City of London; what you really need in healthcare is collaboration rather than competition.

The internal market was introduced on the premise that the NHS is a monolithic bureaucracy, encased in red tape and stifled by centralisation. In other words, the public sector is inefficient and the private sector brings innovation. In fact, as a direct result of these reforms, NHS costs rose substantially. This is largely due to increased numbers of administrative and managerial staff.

A 2005 study by a team at York University demonstrated this.[1]

Administrative costs rose from 5% in the mid 1970s to 14% in 2003 mainly due to internal market operations.

Around 10% of the NHS budget or £10 billion a year is therefore spent on running an internal market.

In fact, this study was commissioned by the Department of Health but hushed up, leading Parliament's Health Select Committee to state that they were 'dismayed' and 'appalled':

'The suspicion must remain that the DoH [Department of Health] does not want the full story to be revealed'.

Recent reforms have added to these costs. The Health & Social Care Act could push these **administrative costs to 30%, which is similar to the US.**

This experience of market-based reforms has been borne out in other countries. A minority report from an NHS working group highlighted evidence from international experts of soaring administrative costs in New Zealand, Canada, Australia and Germany. In the case of Germany, these costs have soared by 63% from 1992 to 2003 now accounting for 20% of the health budget.[2]

Step Two:
Introduce Public-Private Partnerships

When Thatcher was asked what her greatest achievement had been, what was her answer?

a) Falklands War
b) Smashing the miners' strike and deunionisation
c) Privatisation of public utilities
d) The big bang deregulation of the City of London

None of these. It was... NEW LABOUR!

In the same speech, Ken Clarke, ever the good sport, was gracious enough to acknowledge the debt owed to New Labour for perpetuating the marketisation doctrines of Thatcherism. In fact, New Labour had pledged to abolish the internal market but then went full throttle in the opposite direction. New Labour's NHS Plan (2000) and NHS Improvement Plan (2004) resulted in the internal market expanding into an extensive market. This was again based on the premise that the private sector would introduce choice and competition as well as cutting costs.

In 2000, a 'concordat' between the NHS and private health firms paved the way for the provision of elective care and diagnostic tests, paid for by the NHS. This concordat facilitated private companies becoming permanent providers of treatment to NHS patients.

For example, when your GP requests an ultrasound or MRI scan, there is a good chance that a private company is being paid by the NHS to carry this out. Again, when your GP refers you to an outpatient clinic to see a specialist, this may be run by a private company. In theory, this sounds like a good idea.

Tim Evans, who negotiated the concordat on behalf of the

private sector, looked forward **'to a time when the NHS would simply be a kitemark attached to the institutions and activities of a system of purely private providers'.**[1]

These public-private partnerships would take many shapes, the first of which were Independent Sector Treatment Centres (ISTC). ISTCs served as the entry point for the private sector and were intended to 'unbundle' the high-volume, low-risk, lucrative NHS work, such as cataracts and knee and hip replacements. In so doing, they would reduce waiting times. The concept may have been simple enough but the reality was messy.[2]

As the British Medical Association (BMA) has shown, ISTC contracts were paid an average of 12% more for each patient than the NHS tariff cost.[3] These sweeteners are often used in the outsourcing of public services to attract the private sector. They were also paid for a pre-determined number of cases—in bulk— regardless of whether procedures were carried out or not. To take one example, **'Netcare did not perform nearly 40% of the work it had been contracted to do', receiving £35 million for patients it never treated.**[4]

As of 2010, an overall average of just 85% of contracted activity was delivered. They ended up costing £5.6 billion over 5 years, yet by 2008 barely exceeded 2% of 8.6 million elective procedures.

Bringing in the private sector did not cut costs. It increased costs to the detriment of the NHS and patients, with only the private sector benefiting.

On top of this, clinical complications and legal costs were covered by the NHS. Yet more sugar-coating. There have also been repeated concerns about quality of care. Nevertheless, ISTCs were widened into the Extended Choice Network, which comprised 149 privately-run facilities by 2009.

Outsourced services are allowed to use the NHS logo meaning that patients are in the dark about who exactly provides their care. It was win-win for ISTC contractors and lose-lose for the NHS and patients. So if you are having an elective procedure or operation in the future, find out if it is being performed by a private company.

ISTCs were small fry compared to Private Finance Initiatives (PFIs). New Labour expanded PFIs, originally dreamt up under John Major, to build *and run* infrastructure projects. PFI schemes were used to build roads, schools, prisons and hospitals. PFI hospitals made up the biggest chunk. These projects were put out to tender to PFI consortia of bankers, construction firms and facilities management companies. This kept the money off the treasury's books and reduced the costs of government borrowing. Again, it was too good to be true. The completed PFI projects have been leased back to the government (or in the case of PFI hospitals to NHS trusts) with repayments, usually over 25 to 30 years, at high interest rates (some over 70%). Repayments are indexed so that they increase every year, even when the income of NHS trusts is falling. The Conservatives are fond of drawing analogies between the economy and a household budget; so think of PFI as a mortgage… a hideously expensive mortgage, which ends up bankrupting the family!

The bill for hospitals alone is projected to rise above £79 billion. This exceeds the original capital cost (i.e. actual value) of £11.4 billion seven-fold.[5]

PFIs came with strings attached in which 'facilities mainte-nance' was also subcontracted out. For example, if you need to change a plug socket or a light bulb, only a specific contractor is allowed to do this.[6] A *Daily Telegraph* investigation flagged up several examples for the edification of the general public but this one really stands out:

One hospital was charged £52,000 for a job, which should have cost £750.[7]

If you wanted to think up a way to bleed the NHS dry then you would struggle to do better than PFI. Is it any wonder then that **more than half of NHS hospitals are now in deficit and potentially in danger of going bust? It is estimated that as many as three quarters of all hospitals could be in deficit in 2015.**[8]

One of the main factors behind this is PFI, although this is not usually mentioned.

The total PFI tab for the taxpayer stands at £301 billion for infrastructure projects with a capital worthof £54.7 billion.

That's a difference of £246 billion.

Just think what you could do with this money?

Well it would pay for all the nurses (there are just under 350,000) in the NHS for 10 years.

Plus all 40,000 consultants for 10 years.

Plus all 40,000 GPs for 10 years.[9]

Still £67 billion to burn.

Well there are 18,000 surgeons in England. It costs around £400,000 to train a surgeon (surgeons and fighter pilots are the two most expensive professions to train so I'm told). So the next generation or two of surgeons i.e. another 18,000 would cost around £7 billion.[10]

Plus 80 state of the art hospitals (based on the estimated cost of the new Papworth hospital—the national heart and lung transplant centre—at £165 million).[11]

And pay for chemotherapy and radiotherapy for a million cancer patients (at £35,000 each).[12]

If you wanted to keep it simple then the PFI drain would cover the entire NHS budget for over 2 years.

And with the leftover change, you could cover Wayne Rooney's £300,000 a week salary should Manchester United ever require a government bailout! And even George Osborne's first-class train fares (in view of his tendency for fare-dodging) until the next election.

PFIs and ISTCs are just two examples of how the private sector and a few really high-net-worth individuals have siphoned off public money.

I was born at the Queen Elizabeth hospital in Birmingham. My father has been under their excellent care for many years. It has been rebuilt as a PFI hospital with the original cost at £627 million but repayments will reach £2.58 billion.[13] This begs the question: how many other patients could receive fantastic NHS care for this money?

I did my GP training at the Royal London Hospital, which is part of Barts Health trust. This is the largest trust in the country and accordingly has the most expensive PFI scheme, which is one of Innisfree's flagship projects. Innsifree is the biggest player in the PFI market. The original capital cost (i.e. actual value) of the Barts Health PFI was £1.1 billion (around £1 million per bed) but will end up costing £7.1 billion by 2049.[14]

£6 billion will go to the PFI consortium Skanska Innisfree and partners. Barts Health are paying £100 million a year in interest before they even see a patient.[15] That's £3 billion, just in interest, over 30 years. Imagine what you could do for healthcare in East London with this money.

So it's not exactly surprising that Barts Health have declared that they are in dire financial straits.

The Princess Royal Hospital in Bromley was another Innisfree gift to the taxpayer. It will cost the NHS ten times what it is worth—that's £1.2 billion.[16] It's the main reason why South London Healthcare Trust went bust in 2012. Norfolk and Norwich University Hospital is another PFI part-owned by Innisfree. A few years into the contract, the PFI owners refinanced it, raising their annual rate of return from 16 to 60%.

There are many more Innisfree PFI timebombs detonating up and down the country—19 in total. The healthcare of people in all these areas is jeopardised just so that Chief Executive David Metter and his total of 25 employees—yes that's right 25—can make a killing![17] The *Daily Telegraph* describes him as the 'the man, who owns 28 hospitals and a motorway'. At the last count, one might add.

Apparently there's no money left. Unless you are someone like **Metter, who took home £8.6 million in pay and dividends in 2010.**

Money that could have been used to treat patients, pay for more NHS staff and build more hospitals instead of cuts, sacking staff and closing hospitals. This is why Conservative MP Edward Leigh, chair of a Treasury Committee report on PFI, described it as the unacceptable face of capitalism.

The insidious encroachment of the private sector into the NHS had thus far been a salubrious warning of the unchartered waters that lay ahead. Or so you might have thought...

So the next time some minister or policy wonk bangs on about the NHS being unaffordable, it's worth remembering the scandalous cost of PFI. The toxic PFI debt has led to hospital mergers with consequent bed reductions, staff lay-offs and service closures. These mergers will be followed by the final 'wave of closures in the run-up to privatisation and franchising out'.[18] As Allyson Pollock astutely points out, the great irony is that PFI was once hailed as the largest hospital-building programme ever; in fact, it is the largest NHS hospital closure programme.

You bet there's an alternative.

One begins to discern a pattern here. Could it be that those advocating bringing in the private sector do not have the interests of the NHS at heart? You would imagine that the case for terminating PFI, in the public interest, even if it means buying out or renegotiating the contracts, is a strong one. The National Audit Office recommended that the government should have the power to cancel contracts, which are not providing value for money.[19] In fact, one hospital has done just that by buying out its PFI contract—West Park Hospital in Darlington (expected to save £14 million). However, this is not feasible for larger PFI contracts, such as Barts Health, without the backing of government.

The effective renationalisation of Network Rail and the London Underground Public-Private Partnership upgrade provide precedents.[20] However, this government does not have the political will to do this. They believe in the ideology of neoliberalism and are against the role of state provision.

In fact, the Treasury has been the midwife to PFI2—a rebranding exercise, which sounds like a summer blockbuster sequel. Unfortunately it will be hospitals not movie villains, which will be blown up as a result. It is likely that PFI2—with higher rates of return for investors—will prove to be more expensive than the original PFI.[21]

Step Three:
Facilitate the Corporate Takeover

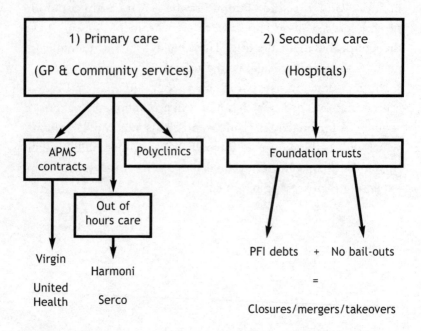

1) Primary care:

The introduction of **Alternative Provider Medical Services (APMS)** contracts meant that Primary Care Trusts (PCTs) could commission care from companies employing salaried GPs rather than traditional contracts with GPs themselves. Amongst the winners were UnitedHealth (more on which later), Atos (to which the government outsourced the controversial fitness tests for incapacity and other benefits) and Virgin.

The corporate takeover of **Out-of-Hours Care (OOH)** saw companies like Harmoni, Serco and Take Care Now win contracts to provide OOH care. Harmoni has been the leader in this field, quietly hoovering up whole swathes of OOH care nationwide.

2) Secondary care:

Foundation trusts were introduced from 2003. This empty-sounding label essentially converted hospitals into semi-independent businesses with financial and other freedoms.

New GP and consultant contracts were negotiated in 2003-4. The GP contract appeared to be a major triumph. It made OOH care optional and led to increased pay for GP partners matching hospital consultant salaries. However, in the long run, it proved to be a significant own goal. Firstly, there was a backlash against GPs from Parliament, the CBI and the media, typified by the *Daily Mail's* coruscating front pages slamming 'super GPs earning £250,000'. Never mind the distortion of this applying only to a tiny number of GPs and that the Department of Health (DoH) had anticipated the majority of GPs opting out of OOH.[1]

Harmoni has been beset by allegations of cost-cutting, inadequate staffing and sub-standard care, most recently as part of *The Guardian's* NHS Plc series. Serco and Take Care Now have also been implicated in similar controversies. **On at least one night, it is alleged that Serco had only one or two GPs covering most (if not all) of Cornwall. It was also claimed that Serco had falsified data to meet targets.**[2] A parliamentary report, by the Public Accounts Committee, highlighted this and accused the company of bullying employees. This contract has now been terminated. Serco has been dogged by scandals in recent times. *The Independent* revealed that Britain's largest pathology services provider Viapath—established as a joint venture by Serco in partnership with Guy's and St Thomas' Hospitals—has been **overcharging for diagnostic tests**. It is estimated that the amount could be as high as £1 million in 2012 alone. There have also been safety concerns and pay cuts leading to loss of experienced staff.[3] If this all sounds familiar, that's because it is. Serco have been **under investigation by the Serious Fraud Office** for overcharging the government for electronic tagging of prisoners. Astonishingly, Serco continues to make profits from taxpayer money. 2013-14 NHS figures show that it was paid £10 million. G4S—also plagued by scandal—took £3.5 million.

None of this should surprise us, as private companies only have one legal obligation, which is to their shareholders. In other words, their aim is to maximise profits usually through cutting staff and other costs. In this sense, the private sector can be seen to be more efficient.

The story behind these outfits is even more intriguing. *The Guardian* exposé describes how Harmoni was formed as a joint venture between the ECI private equity group and a GP co-operative.[4] Its annual turnover mushroomed from £3 million to £100 million. It was then sold to Care UK, which is owned by another private equity group—Bridgepoint—for £48 million. ECI took £20 million and the GP owners of the co-op became million-aires. We'll come back to the links between Care UK and the Tories later.

Virgin Assura claim to have a network of 30 GP partnerships with over 1,500 GPs looking after 3 million patients. Astonishing figures when one is accustomed to thinking of the NHS as an impervious and timeless institution rather than one that is fragmenting as we speak. As of July 2010, 227 GP surgeries and health centres were privately run, with 9 firms including Care UK, holding ten or more contracts. Incidentally, BMA (the doctors' union) negotiators set up a company by the name of Concordia Health and rapidly secured several APMS contracts.

What about the rest of primary care? In 2006-7, the government commissioned Lord Darzi to look into reconfiguring NHS services for the future. The brainchild of his report was the concept of a polyclinic. Polyclinics are large GP centres, with a wide variety of services that you might expect to find at a local hospital, including maternity care, mental health services, multidisciplinary teams, diagnostics and even specialist care. In fact, they seemed like such a good idea that they were rolled out nationwide, with the aim of having one polyclinic in every Primary Care Trust. There was just one snag. **Polyclinics, like everything else in this story, were inextricably linked to privatisation—they were on the whole to be privately financed and run.**

The running costs proved to be hideously expensive and, ultimately, their fate was ignominious. Although polyclinics were wound up, they have been the progenitors to a second wave of GP-led health centres based on APMS contracts. This rebranding was a misnomer obscuring their corporate nature.[5]

With general practice under this all-out assault, what of hospital care? From 2002 onwards, the DoH fixated on the model of **integrated care** utilised by Kaiser Permanente—a large California-based Health Maintenance Organisation (HMO), where the doctors are jointly partners and salaried employees. In a nutshell, integrated care is about the management of long term conditions through alternative systems and pathways to traditional methods (i.e. in hospital). This mainly involves managing these conditions in the community and keeping expensive, hospital care to a minimum. Again, not a bad idea in principle.

However, it is debatable as to whether integrated care is cheaper. Health economist Professor Maynard has cited many integrated care evaluations, including by the DoH, which demonstrate no savings.[6] In 2006, the NHS National Leadership Network produced a document stating that integrated care is not just about the shift of hospital care towards the community but the reconfiguration of NHS infrastructure. There would be a radical reduction in the number of NHS hospitals with the development of new facilities to house integrated care services 'decoupled' from the NHS. This would dovetail nicely with an expansion of the private sector. In other words, **there would be**

shrinkage of NHS-provided services with private ownership as the new norm.

In fact, England has one of the lowest numbers of hospitals based on population, coming in below Poland, Czech Republic, Estonia, Mexico and Korea.[7] It is important to bear this in mind when considering the current debate about closing down smaller hospitals and centralising services into large centres. This may be sensible for highly specialised areas like trauma or stroke care. However, it is not necessarily best for common in-patient admissions (such as pneumonia), outpatient clinics and maternity care. The shift towards community care also requires the allocation of resources. In fact, the opposite has been happening with chronic-underinvestment in general practice. All in all, the evidence base for these reconfigurations is shaky. It is likely that vested interests see service redesign as the pre-requisite to privatisation.

'Kaiser beacon' pilots have already been trialed, and integrated care organisations have started springing up, such as Principia Partners in Health. Circle—the first private company to run an NHS hospital (Hinchingbrooke Hospital)—are very much based on the Kaiser model of co-ownership. However, this experiment has ended ignominiously with Circle's involvement deemed unsustainable and the hospital rated inadequate and put into special measures. **As a disclaimer, it should be mentioned that Kaiser are infamous for 'dumping' patients in downtown Los Angeles.** Yes, literally dumping patients in hospital gowns when their insurance policies have expired. There are over 50 such alleged cases. Not exactly the kind of ethos we should import over here.

When I was a junior doctor, I worked at Guy's and St Thomas' Hospital, which is a foundation trust, but I had no idea what this meant. Foundation trust status gave hospitals greater independence. For example, hospitals can make business partnerships. **The flip side is that foundation trusts are allowed to 'go bust'** as they are no longer eligible to be bailed out by the DoH. In this event, Monitor (the NHS regulator) can invite another trust to take over or alternatively leave the hospital to close. This was a paradigm shift as it forced hospitals to prioritise the bottom line over patient care.

A system of payment by results was also introduced, which meant hospitals being 'paid per completed treatment and not a lump sum for a given total'. These payments are based on 'a national tariff of fixed prices, adjusted for the seriousness of each category'.[8] Both foundation trusts and payment by results have increased administration and transaction costs. Transaction costs include: 'advertising, negotiating, contracting, invoicing, billing, auditing, monitoring contracts, collecting information, resolving disputes both in courts and out'.[9]

Many hospitals have rushed to attain foundation trust status. They have therefore needed to balance their books, which has often meant cutting frontline staff. **This was one of the main factors behind the Mid Staffs scandal, involving the deaths of hundreds of patients at Stafford Hospital in Staffordshire.** Poor care was not actually due to an uncaring ethos as has been suggested. It was often down to the lack of sufficient nursing staff on the wards as the Francis Inquiry concluded. In other words, this was yet another example of how market-based reforms have led to worse outcomes for the NHS and patients. Ironically, Mid Staffs then spent more on adequate staffing, went into deficit and was deemed unsustainable.

Foundation trust status may have seemed attractive but hospital bosses did not anticipate the current climate of cuts (including cuts to hospital tariffs) combined with mounting PFI debts. **As a result, tens of trusts up and down the country are running into the red. More than a third of NHS trusts in acute deficit are hospitals built under PFI.**[10]

Step Four:
Install a Revolving Door

How did all of this happen? The short answer is the **revolving door**. Two former secretaries of state for health (Milburn and Hewitt) and one minister for health (Lord Warner) packed their bags after discharging their public duties and headed for the lucrative pastures of post-Westminster retirement in the private sector.

As Colin Leys and Stewart Player have pointed out, **Alan Milburn**, Secretary of State for Health 1999-2003, went on to become an adviser to Bridgepoint Capital (a private equity firm involved in financing Alliance Medical and Care UK), Lloyds Pharmacy, Covidien (medical suppliers) and Pepsico. **Patricia Hewitt** was Secretary of State for Health 2005-7. Hewitt then became adviser to private equity company Cinven (which bought Bupa's chain of 25 private hospitals) and was paid £60,000 for 18 days' work a year. She was also a 'special consultant' to Alliance Boots at an annual salary of £40,000 and a non-executive director of BT at a salary of £60,000. In the cash for access scandal, she was caught by Channel 4's Dispatches offering to use her contacts 'on behalf of the imaginary clients of a fictitious US lobbying firm for £3,000 a day'.[1]

Further down the pyramid, **Simon Stevens,** Blair's senior health policy advisor, who went to work for UnitedHealth (as an Executive Vice President), eventually came back to haunt us (through said revolving door) as no less than the chief executive of the NHS. The former *British Medical Journal* editor Richard Smith also went to work for UnitedHealth.

The revolving door turns smoothly in both directions. Management consultants from McKinsey, KPMG, Deloitte and Atos, to name a few, infiltrated the top tiers of the DoH. A similar pattern emerges across NHS management. This is how the health policy community was hijacked.

NHS England's Deputy Chief Executive Ian Dalton left for BT in February 2013. While Dalton ran their 'global health division, BT received £18 million in contracts from NHS England'.[2] Monitor Chief Executive David Bennett 'spent 18 years with McKinsey before becoming chief policy adviser to Tony Blair and head of the Prime Minister's Strategy Unit'. We'll come back to other links between Monitor and McKinsey. Penny Dash was head of strategy at the DoH before joining McKinsey. Whilst there, she developed the NHS Plan 2000, which expanded the internal market. She also co-founded the Cambridge Health Network, which aims to bring NHS and private healthcare leaders together. Tom Kibasi rejoined McKinsey after two years out as senior policy adviser to former NHS Chief Executive David Nicholson.[3]

In 2009, it was estimated that spending on management consultants alone was upwards of £300 million a year.[4] Andrew Lansley, former Conservative health secretary, stated that he was 'staggered by the scale of the expenditure'. However, since the Coalition came to power, management consultant fees have doubled to £640 million.[5] It seems that austerity, like taxes, only applies to the little people.

The results of this management consultancy culture have included PFIs and Connecting for Health. The latter is the **national NHS IT programme—recommended by McKinsey and run by a consultant from Deloitte—which is largely non-operational at a haemorrhaging cost of £20 billion**, equivalent to the entire efficiency savings (based on a set of 120 PowerPoint slides prepared by McKinsey) the NHS was asked to make between 2011 and 2014.

However, some of these costs could have been mitigated. Richard Granger (Director-General of the NHS National Programme for IT) did not charge Accenture £1 billion as permitted by the contract when they withdrew from the project in 2006. Instead they were only fined £63 million. Granger's next job was with Andersen Consulting (later Accenture).[6]

The revolving door spins into Downing Street. **Nick Seddon** is Cameron's new health advisor. Here are openDemocracy and Social Investigations on his background:

> 'Seddon's last role was as deputy director of "Reform" — a free market think-tank extensively funded by healthcare and insurance companies. **He has openly called for an end to the NHS as we know it, and promoted the idea of an insurance-based system.**... A *Telegraph* article by Seddon highlighted a Reform report, titled "It can be done", which praised the increased involvement of private companies in running hospitals in Spain and Germany'.

No prizes for guessing why Seddon is in favour of all this. He was previously head of communications at Circle, which you will recall became the first private company to run an NHS hospital at Hinchingbrooke.

This is what he had to say on Clinical Commissioning Groups (CCGs): 'There is no evidence to suggest that they [GPs] have the skills needed, which makes it unlikely that they'll be any good at trying to make hospitals improve what they do and cut their costs...'.

However, CCGs could be used as the basis to move towards a 'mixed funding insurance model. **The £80 billion budget could be allocated to insurers in professional alliances with GP groups... those who can afford to would be encouraged to contribute more towards their care packages'.**[7]

This kind of remark is very useful. Every now and again, there is an unguarded comment from those in the know, devoid of all spin. Seddon is clearly referring to healthcare insurance. And this is exactly how we should view CCGs—as insurance pools. The concept of a National Health Service has been replaced by insurance pools allocating the central government funding stream (increasingly to private companies) with tighter criteria, leading to greater rationing of treatment.

Over 200 parliamentarians have recent past or present financial interests in companies involved in private healthcare—147 Lords and 73 MPs—according to Social Investigations. *The Mirror* listed 70 MPs with links to private healthcare in an article in November 2014.[8] No surprise then that they are selling off our NHS.

Private companies with financial links to Conservative politicians have won contracts worth £1.5 billion, according to research by the largest trade union, Unite. The most notorious example of this is the former health secretary and architect of the reforms, Andrew Lansley, receiving a donation of £21,000 from Caroline Nash, the wife of John Nash. At the time, John Nash was the chairman of private healthcare company Care UK.[9]

The notion of a boundary between the public and private sectors, which should be policed in the public interest, has long been expunged. There is certainly something rotten in the state of the NHS but, contrary to what the right-wing media and the Conservatives espouse, it is most definitely not NHS care or staff. And when the stench is so overwhelming then you have to call it what it is—Corruption with a capital C; the kind of corruption normally associated with mafia states and banana republics.

Step Five:
Organise a Great Big Sell Off

Here are some of the winners according to Colin Leys and Stewart Player in their book, *The Plot Against the NHS*:

- Private healthcare companies, both British, such as Care UK and Tribal, and international, such as Netcare (a South African hospital chain, which opened several ISTCs and bought a large chain of private hospitals) and UnitedHealth (GP followed by commissioning contracts on behalf of CCGs)
- NHS IT contracts e.g. the Connecting for Health (CfH) fiasco, NHS statistics Dr Foster, NHS choices system (Capita)
- Big Seven companies in hospital cleaning, catering, laundry (with annual revenues totalling £2 billion)
- PFI consortia (£7.1 billion due in 5 years 2010/11-2015/16 — corresponding to almost half the savings the NHS is expected to make in the same period)

So who really are the benefactors of this hidden hand? The scale of the 'marketiser's network', as labelled by corporate watchdog Spinwatch, is vast. Let's start with Serco—a *Guardian* profile described it as 'the biggest company you've never heard of':

'As well as five British prisons and the tags attached to over 8,000 English and Welsh offenders, Serco sees to two immigration removal centres.... You'll also see its logo on the Docklands Light Railway and Woolwich ferry, and is a partner in both Liverpool's Merseyrail network, and the Northern Rail franchise.... Serco runs school inspections in parts of England, speed cameras all over the UK, and the National Nuclear Laboratory, based at the Sellafield site in Cumbria. It also holds the contracts for the management of the UK's ballistic missile early warning system on the Yorkshire moors.... But even this is only a fraction of the story. Among their scores of roles across the planet, Serco is responsible for air traffic control in the United Arab Emirates, parking-meter services in Chicago, driving tests in Ontario, and an immigration detention centre on Christmas Island'.[1]

The *Daily Telegraph* puts it bluntly: 'Without Serco, Britain would struggle to go to war'. The parallels with a *New York Times* profile of Lockheed Martin (potentially bidding for NHS contracts) are clear to see:

'Lockheed Martin doesn't run the United States. But it does help run a breathtakingly big part of it. Over the last decade, Lockheed, the nation's largest military contractor, has built a formidable information-technology empire that now stretches from the Pentagon to the post office. It sorts your mail and totals your taxes. It cuts Social Security checks and counts the United States census. It runs space flights and monitors air traffic. To make all that happen, Lockheed writes more computer code than Microsoft'.[2]

The South African company **Netcare** is one of the leading lights in private hospital chains. Netcare has been implicated in illegal kidney transplants with the knowledge of its chief executive, according to South African prosecutors. Although it has denied some of these allegations, it has admitted to receiving £342,000 from an organ trafficking syndicate for assisting with **illegal kidney transplants including from 5 children.**[3]

Next up is UnitedHealth Group, the single largest health carrier in the US and one of the top 20 Fortune 500 US corporations with an annual revenue of $120 billion in 2014.[4] In 2009, their CEO pocketed over $100 million (I would have to work for

1,700 years to earn this sum!). **UnitedHealth** have been repeatedly forced to pay massive fines for **multiple instances of fraud** involving various branches of the US government. The share options scam involving the Department of Health's Channing Wheeler and previous CEO Dr William McGuire led to UnitedHealth being forced to hand back hundreds of millions of dollars to shareholders. The State of **California was seeking nearly $10 billion in fines**, although this has been revised significantly downwards.[5] For companies like UnitedHealth, these fines are loose pocket change. This is just part and parcel of how they do business.

Dr William McGuire's exit compensation is said to have been— wait for it—$1.1 billion. In the United States, healthcare-related fraud is endemic. UnitedHealth has run GP surgeries and is preparing to become one of the major players in commissioning. UnitedHealth has also paid for senior NHS executives to travel to the US to see how the company operates and explore applicability in the UK. It is remarkable that we are opening the door in Britain to these multinationals mired in scandal and fraud. Perhaps this is what Jeremy Hunt means by rediscovering a caring ethos in the NHS. Remember that NHS chief executive Simon Stevens used to work for UnitedHealth, so yet again we shouldn't be too surprised.[6]

And then there is **McKinsey**. The US firm is the largest management consultancy in the world. The *Mail on Sunday* described it as the firm that hijacked the NHS in an exposé revealing how it had lavished NHS regulators, drawn up proposals for the Health & Social Care Act and used access to share information with other clients.[7]

McKinsey's fingerprints are all over NHS reforms. We have already come across Penny Dash, behind the NHS Plan 2000 and the Darzi plans for polyclinics, and Dr David Bennett, former McKinsey director and current Chairman of Monitor. McKinsey produced the 2008 report NHS London and the 2009 financial analysis behind the efficiency savings (cuts of £15-20 billion up to 2014).

In a climate of economic stagnation, corporations are turning to opening the oyster of European public services in order to continue generating massive profits. The NHS alone represents over a staggering £100 billion.

Step Six:
Run a PR Smear Campaign

The relentless anti-NHS smear campaign, run by various sectors of the media, is now escalating, softening up the public in preparation for the introduction of universal health insurance coverage. Certainly the proliferation of private healthcare ads suggests that insurance companies are already licking their lips at this mouthwatering prospect. There is a simple test to establish whether this is indeed a PR campaign. Who runs the NHS? The government of course, stupid. And yet there has been not so much as a murmur of protest in defense of this all-out assault on *its* NHS.

There has been neither a democratic mandate nor an evidence-base for these reforms. Factsheets on the DoH website summarise the government's case for change.[1] This is largely premised upon affordability (notably in the context of the current state of the nation's finances) and modernising the NHS to improve standards. If you believe what you read in the papers then these arguments would seem utterly persuasive. There have been consistent doubts cast, in the media, on the affordability of the NHS and on the standard of care it provides. This aids the government's agenda of promoting reform but the real data undermines this case.

IS THE NHS AFFORDABLE?

This is one of the key questions. I repeatedly hear colleagues and friends ask, 'But where will the money come from?'

John Appleby, the Chief Economist at the King's Fund, has largely dismantled the case that the NHS is unaffordable in the pages of the *British Medical Journal*.[2] We'll let the charts do the talking....

Here are the Organisation for Economic Co-operation and Development (OECD) figures in health spending:

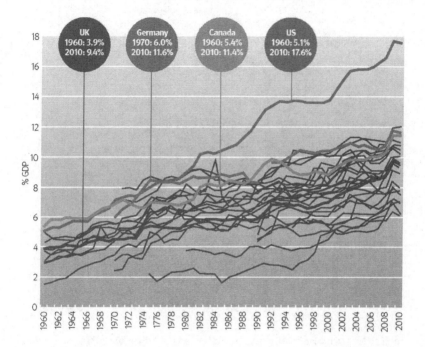

Approaching £1 in £10 of its economic wealth, in 2010 the UK devoted more than twice the share of GDP to public plus private healthcare spending as it did in 1960. The US spent around 5% of GDP on healthcare in 1960. Today it is nudging 18%, and in total the US spends almost the same on health as all other countries in the OECD put together. Germany, France, and the Netherlands now spend around €1 in €8 on healthcare.

Reproduced with permission of the author John Appleby from 'Rises in healthcare spending: where will it end?' Published in the *British Medical Journal* (BMJ) in 2012.

Here are the figures for EU-15 countries health spending:

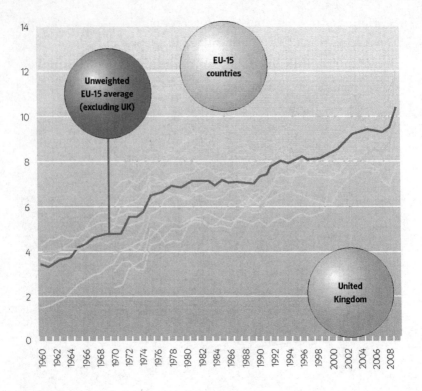

Total healthcare spending of EU-15 countries (Austria, Belgium, Denmark, Finland, France, Germany, Greece, Ireland, Italy, Luxembourg, the Netherlands, Portugal, Spain, Sweden, and UK) as a proportion of GDP, 1960-2008. Unweighted average = sum of percentages/number of countries submitting data in each year.

Reproduced with permission of the author John Appleby from 'Can we afford the NHS in future?' Published 12/7/11 BMJ 2011;343:d4321

In a 2011 paper, John Appleby cites an article Andrew Lansley wrote in the *Telegraph*, in which he stated that by 2030, 'If things carry on unchanged, this would mean real terms health spending more than doubling to £230 billion' and that 'this is something we simply cannot afford'.[3]

Healthcare spending is at around 9.3% of GDP. As Appleby

surmises, based on projections, £230 billion as a proportion of GDP in 2030 will amount to 10.9%. 'Adding private spending on healthcare to NHS spend (to enable better comparison with other countries), total spend in 2030 could be around 12.4% of GDP '.

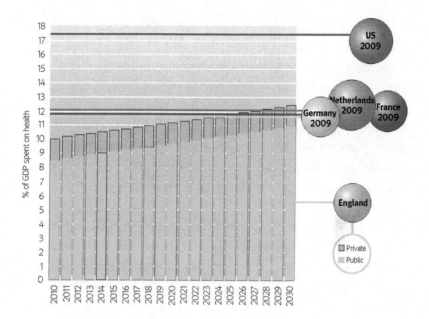

Possible future English healthcare spending 2010-30 as proportion of GDP. Figures are hypothetical and assume English private spending is 1.5% of GDP.

Reproduced with permission of the author John Appleby from 'Can we afford the NHS in future? Published 12/7/11 BMJ 2011;343:d4321

As Appleby concludes, 'this would make England the highest spending country in the OECD bar the US—but only assuming no other country increased its spending on healthcare. Even in 2009, seven of the EU-15 countries spent over 10% of GDP on healthcare. The highest spender—the Netherlands—devoted 12% of its GDP to healthcare'.

In fact, UK spending on healthcare is less than all other G7 countries apart from Italy, which spends the same, according to the Office for National Statistics (ONS). On current projections, UK spending could even fall to 6% of GDP by 2021 (due to cuts) according to the King's Fund think-tank.[4]

In summary, there are two key points. First, rising healthcare costs are a fact across the world.[5] Second, **the NHS is one of the most inexpensive healthcare systems** in the developed world. We have already seen how market-based reforms—such as the internal market, foundation trusts and payment by results— actually increase costs. Bringing in the private sector—in the form of PFIs or ISTCs to name two examples—has generally lined the pockets of corporations whilst producing worse outcomes for the NHS and patients, not to mention running hospitals into the ground.

Market-based healthcare systems tend to be more expensive than the NHS. In the 1960s, the economist and Nobel laureate Kenneth Arrow demonstrated that the normal rules of the market do not apply to healthcare. The US system is the best example of this, with healthcare costs going through the roof. This is because classical market forces do not exert the usual control and do not regulate supply and demand. Physicians are paid through a fee-for-service system, which basically means that the more they do, the more they are paid. Likewise, hospitals and laboratories aim to increase their services to maximise profits. Pharmaceuticals and medical manufacturers also promote their products aggressively. Combine all of this with minimal regulation of prices, add in for-profit private insurance plans with some giant insurance corporations, and you have a system in which costs are out of control, driven by profit incentives and not by medical need. Unsurprisingly, this set-up encourages gaming of the system with fraudulent billing and inflated charges accounting for a significant amount of healthcare fraud.[6]

The question should not be whether we can afford the NHS

but what kind of healthcare system do we want?

An NHS England document—'The NHS belongs to the people'—projects a £30 billion funding gap by 2020.[7] Hence Professor Malcolm Grant, NHS England chairman, airing that **post-2015, NHS user charges would need to be considered**. This is the man who has been on record as saying 'I don't use the NHS'.[8] Migrant user charges have been mooted introducing a charging mechanism into the NHS. However, there is a simple reason why we do not have user charges. Successive governments have undertaken major reviews of NHS funding, including Sir Derek Wanless' 2002 report for the Treasury. They have all concluded that central taxation is the most efficient and fairest system.[9] Ministers handed back a £2.2 billion underspend from the NHS budget to the Treasury in 2013 following an underspend of over £1.4 billion similarly handed back in 2012.[10]

The Nuffield Trust think-tank produced a paper, 'A Decade of Austerity?' projecting that the efficiency savings should be extended.[11] The question appears to be rhetorical. Efficiency savings have now been extended until 2021 and **could possibly reach £50 billion** by 2019-20, according to the DoH.[12,13]

On international comparisons, NHS performance is good. **The US-based Commonwealth Fund's large study of 20,000 patients in 11 industrialised countries found the NHS to be almost the least costly and to have almost the best levels of access.**

'Other countries not only spent more per head but also charged patients directly, reducing equality of access. Only Switzerland reported faster access to care but Switzerland also spent some 35 per cent more per head than the UK. Only New Zealand spent less per head, but one in seven said they skipped hospital visits because of cost. In the US, which spent almost twice as much per head as the UK, one in three Americans avoided seeking care because of cost'.[14]

This report was updated in 2014 by the Commonwealth Fund finding that, **'The United Kingdom ranks first overall, scoring highest on quality, access and efficiency'.**[15] But you will not have seen this headline carried by many newspapers: NHS BEST HEALTH SYSTEM IN THE WORLD! On the other hand, the US was castigated as the worst of the 11 countries despite putting the most money into health.[16]

The OECD's *Health at a Glance* (2011), one of the most respected sources of international comparisons, corroborated this picture of the NHS being amongst the best in the world. According to their head of health Mark Pearson, 'The UK is one of the best performers in the world.' The DoH grudgingly conceded that the NHS is performing well for patients. The OECD also emphasised that the NHS has cut heart attack deaths by two-thirds since 1980. Less than 5% of adults had diabetes in 2010, contrasting with 10% in the United States.[17]

This is not to say that the NHS does not have weaknesses. As with any system in the world, there is room for improvement, including mortality rates in certain types of cancer. There are also more avoidable hospital admissions for asthma in the UK than the average in the OECD.

In recent years, there have been a number of scandals involving hospital care. Whilst the media is very good at exposing NHS deficiencies, there is only glib analysis of the factors behind this. *The Guardian* managed to run a double page story on the financial troubles of Barts Health, with PFI mentioned as an afterthought.[18] You may recall that we are talking about a £6 billion funding gap generated by its PFI. Quite an omission! Hospitals are operating in a climate of stealth cuts and massive PFI debts leading them to cut frontline staff and divert money away from patient care. As a result, delivery of care has been compromised. These stories present the NHS in a bad light without any explanation.

Take the A&E crisis splashed across the front pages every winter. The take-home message seems to be that the NHS is creaking at the seams and can no longer take the strain. The reality behind the A&E crisis is that it has largely been manufactured due to long-standing problems. For starters, a quarter of walk-in centres have been closed since 2010.[19] This is compounded by **a reduction in bed numbers of over 50% since 1987-8**—from nearly 300,000 down to just 135,000.[20] Britain now has one of the lowest numbers of beds in all of Europe. In fact, hospitals are spending millions buying up increased bed capacity at private hospital chains run by the likes of BMI and Spire.[21] The same companies are bidding for NHS work and are often owned by large private equity firms. This is a case of NHS budgets being simultaneously squeezed on more than one front.

At the same time, there has been a steep decline in the provision of social care, whilst the elderly population and demand have both increased. This means that elderly patients cannot be discharged safely and they end up 'bed-blocking', which therefore has a knock-on effect. In October 2014, there were a record total of 96,564 bed days—when a patient stays in a hospital bed overnight—taken up by patients fit to leave but who could not be discharged due to lack of social care support. In August 2010, there were just 55,332 bed days lost.[22] This is certainly a scenario familiar to every junior doctor.

But the problem is getting worse as local councils tighten eligibility criteria due to massive austerity cuts. **The number of elderly and disabled people receiving care at home has been slashed by a third in the past five years.**[23] These patients are thus more likely to end up in A&E. In fact, you cannot separate out the A&E crisis from the historic social care crisis. Long-term residential care was privatised from Thatcher onwards, and by the end of the 1990s free long-term care provided by the NHS had largely been replaced by private sector care homes charging fees.[24]

In view of all of this, it's not exactly surprising that A&Es are struggling to cope.

John Appleby has examined some of the trends in NHS performance in a paper entitled 'Does poor health justify NHS reform?' The official ministerial briefing for the Health & Social Care Bill stated the rate of death from heart disease is double that of France. Age standardised death rate for heart attacks was around 19/100,000 in France and 41/100,000 in the UK. But this is only true comparing just one year (2006) with the country with the lowest death rate for heart attacks in Europe. The UK has had lower levels of spending every year for the past half century than France. OECD spending comparisons show that in 2008, the UK spent 8.7% of its GDP on health compared with 11.2% for France.[25]

The bigger picture is that the UK has experienced the largest fall in deaths from heart attacks, between 1980 and 2006, of any European country.

Jeremy Hunt himself penned an article in *The Guardian* celebrating that, 'patients who have heart surgery in England have a greater chance of survival than in almost any other European country. Since 2005, death rates have halved and are now far lower than the European average'.[26] Why? Because the surgeons decided to collect, analyse and publish their own data with openness leading to greater success. In other words, improvements in the NHS or any public sector organisation can be achieved without recourse to marketisation or privatisation.

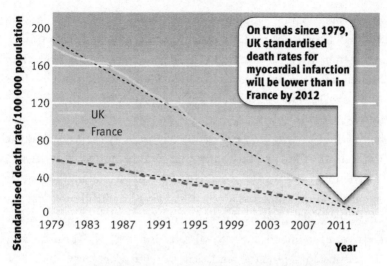

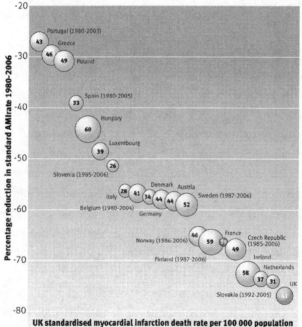

Reproduced with permission of the author John Appleby from 'Does poor health justify NHS reform?' Published 28/1/11 BMJ 2011;342:d566

In the same paper, Appleby goes on to examine cancer data. In the UK, death rates for **lung cancer** in men rose to a peak in 1979. Since then they have steadily fallen and are now **lower than French men**. With regards to **breast cancer** mortality—'since 1989, age standardised death rates per 100,000 in the UK have fallen by 40% to virtually close the gap with France, where they have fallen by just 10%... if trends continue, **it is likely that the UK will have lower death rates than France in just a few years'.**

The Eurocare study—the most comprehensive ongoing study of cancer survival across Europe—often feeds headlines that the UK is the 'sick man of Europe'. Trends from Eurocare actually show improvements in survival rates for the UK—confirmed by the Office for National Statistics. But Eurocare is problematic, with a lag in data several years behind, and patchy coverage (French data cover around 10-15% of people with cancer, whilst UK data cover 100%).

It is also worth bearing in mind that whether one is looking at heart disease or cancer, there are extrinsic factors (such as changing lifestyle patterns or public awareness) not directly connected to the performance of a healthcare system.

And what of the public? As Nicholas Timmins points out, **public satisfaction with the NHS was at its highest ever (as recorded by the British Social Attitudes Survey)** just as the white paper for the Health & Social Care Bill was launched. This is a polling series stretching back to 1983.[27] DoH patient surveys were showing the same thing. **Polling in 2012 showed the NHS to be more popular than even the monarchy.**[28]

We can see that affordability, standards and public satisfaction far from justify a massive upheaval of the NHS. Not only is the cost of the Coalition's reconfiguration estimated at up to £3 billion, but the OECD has stated that such endless reforms are actually holding back the NHS. Mark Pearson, head of health at the OECD points out that 'each reform costs two years of improvements in quality. No country reforms its health service as frequently as the UK'.[29]

Many of the myths and misconceptions surrounding the NHS are often perpetuated by those with a hidden agenda or a vested interest in undermining the NHS. The simple truth is that key establishment figures in the government and media cannot stand the idea of a National Health Service and its public provision of healthcare free at the point of delivery. It is an affront to everything they espouse—that the public sector is inefficient and bureaucratic, that privatisation and markets are always good and that state provision is to be limited as much as possible.

Step Seven:
Legislate for the Dismantling of the NHS

'Just as I was signing off our panel's report on "Delivering real choice" I get sent a copy of the PM's speech announcing he was accepting many of our key recommendations (although we haven't actually given him the report yet!)…'.

Sir Stephen Bubb, who reviewed the role of competition in the NHS for the Health & Social Care Bill.[1]

It was Tony Benn who once predicted a revolution in the streets if the NHS was privatised. On the opposite benches, Nigel Lawson, Thatcher's former chancellor, acknowledged that the NHS is 'the closest thing the English have to a religion'. Therefore the Conservatives knew they could not touch the NHS in the public glare. This had to be undertaken by stealth. Nicholas Timmins has diligently charted this process in *Never Again: The Story of the Health & Social Care Act*.[2] Labour's mantra 'you can't trust the Tories with the NHS' has resonated for many years with the British public. After David Cameron became party leader in 2005, the Tories pulled out all the stops in order to detoxify how they were perceived on the NHS. Cameron, a former Carlton man, knows a thing or two about PR. This was in keeping with the rebranding of the Conservatives as compassionate, repositioning the party towards the centre-ground. The message was 'the NHS is safe in our hands'. The 2010 manifesto promised: 'We are stopping the top-down reconfigurations of NHS services, imposed from Whitehall'.

Only weeks into government, the Tories reverted to form. The mother of all reconfigurations was unveiled in the white paper 'Liberating the NHS' and all hell broke loose.[3] David Nicholson, the NHS chief executive at the time, remarked that the change was so large it was visible from space.[4] The Health & Social Care Bill met with fierce opposition from every conceivable quarter forcing the government to pause for a 'listening exercise'. However, according to *The Guardian* and Social Investigations, **a leaked document revealed that 'the private health lobby worked with Downing Street behind the scenes to ensure that the new legislation went ahead'.**[5]

David Worskett, one of the main lobbyists for the private healthcare industry, wrote in a memo at the time: 'the whole sequence of *Telegraph* articles and editorials on the importance of the Government not going soft on public service reform, including some strong pieces on health, is something I have been orchestrating and working with Reform to bring about'.[6]

The Coalition then embarked on a charm offensive. Cabinet members were wheeled out one after another to placate us with homilies. Not least of all Andrew Lansley, reasserting time and again how passionate he is about the NHS and how cherished it is as a British institution. For the above, read as eulogies. In the words of the doctor and *Daily Telegraph* columnist Max Pemberton, the death warrant had been issued.[7] You know the writing is on the wall when this much praise is being heaped on the NHS by the party, who voted against its establishment and have fought against it ever since. As James Meek put it in the London Review of Books, you can praise something whilst at the same time legislating it out of existence.[8]

The political capital expended has been massive, with public opinion turning against the government handling of the NHS. It is all in keeping with the Coalition's growing reputation for *omnishambles*. However, don't let that fool you. An intriguing question is why the Tories chose to execute this so soon after the election campaign despite repeated avowals to the contrary. The answer may lie in Tony Blair's purported advice to them, which was paraphrased as ramming the bill through as swiftly as possible because the public will have forgotten about it by the time of the next election.[9]

The Coalition emphasised the motifs of the Bill as improving patient choice through competition, empowering doctors and cutting management costs, neatly encapsulated in the euphemistic title of the white paper as 'Liberating the NHS'—all of which is nothing less than a smokescreen for the implementation of free-market reforms. The Health & Social Care document weighs in at a door-stopping 473 pages (tellingly around three times the size of the original 1948 legislation that set up the NHS). But there are only three words that really matter— **ANY QUALIFIED PROVIDER**. This should really be the epitaph on the Coalition's obituary. It means that **competitive tendering of NHS contracts will be opened up to providers from the voluntary and more importantly private sectors**.

Professor Martin McKee, Professor of European Public Health at the London School of Hygiene and Tropical Medicine, dubbed the Act's sheer length and complexity as the Jackson Pollock effect. The Act is said to have been drawn up by a group of corporate lawyers. Professor McKee also compares it to the Schleswig-Holstein question—an arcane complex of diplomatic issues arising in the nineteenth century relating to the two eponymous duchies. British prime-minister Lord Palmerston is reported to have said at the time, 'Only three people... have ever really understood the Schleswig-Holstein business—the Prince Consort, who is dead—a German professor, who has gone mad—and I, who have forgotten all about it'.

In other words, the Bill amounted to deliberate obfuscation that left critics floundering whilst the government got on with the real business of carving up the NHS. Don't take my word for it. Those are the words of Mark Britnell, an NHS manager who became one of the most powerful civil servants in the DoH.

As James Meek has assiduously documented, Britnell went on to work as global head of health for the consultants KPMG.... In 2010 Britnell was interviewed for... a conference in New York: 'In future,' Britnell said, 'the NHS will be a state insurance provider, not a state deliverer... The NHS will be shown no mercy and the best time to take advantage of this will be in the next couple of years'.[10]

The Britnell quote is shocking enough but this was no ordinary conference. Its subject was

'how private companies could take advantage of the vulnerability of healthcare systems in a harsh financial climate'.[11]

This is another of these unguarded and illuminating quotes. The NHS is basically being converted into a state insurance provider like Medicare in the US with CCGs, based on US-managed care organisations, acting as healthcare insurers.

That Britnell was a serious candidate for the most important position in the NHS—the chief executive designate of the NHS Commissioning Board—is a damning indictment and helps explain how we got into this mess in the first place. The position eventually went to the incumbent NHS Chief Executive David Nicholson, who fawningly described the reforms as 'really, really revolutionary'.[12] Britnell has since told the *British Medical Journal* that he is keen to come back to the NHS.

So what does the Act do? According to the BMA:

- The Act places duties on the Secretary of State for Health to promote a comprehensive health service in England.
- The Act enables the Secretary of State to set priorities for the NHS through a mandate for the NHS Commissioning Board.
- The Act also establishes Clinical Commissioning Groups

(CCGs) to be responsible for commissioning local services.[13]

All of these sound perfectly anodyne until you decipher the legalese. This is what Allyson Pollock, David Price and Peter Roderick have done in the *British Medical Journal*. Firstly, the Act severs the duty of the Health Secretary to provide a national health service by devolving this to CCGs. CCGs, unlike Primary Care Trusts, will not have to provide health services for everyone living in their area but only those on the patient lists of GPs. This is an important distinction and allows **exclusion of patients**. There are other exclusionary criteria. CCGs can also decide on what services will be free at the point of delivery. The legislation states that they have the power to determine what is **'appropriate as part of the health service'**. Vague indeed. The only legal requirement for CCGs is to provide ambulance services and emergency care. This means that there will be increased rationing, which fits in with the concept of CCGs as insurance pools ultimately able to exclude the poorest and sickest from coverage.

The authors conclude that:

> **The Act legislates for 'reductions in government funded health services as a consequence of decisions made independently of the secretary of state by a range of bodies.... [It fails] to make clear who is ultimately responsible for people's health services... creates new powers for charging [and]... signals the basis for a shift from a mainly tax financed health service to one in which patients may have to pay for services currently free at point of delivery'.**[14]

Monitor will be the economic regulator for all NHS funded services. It has many roles, including the prevention of anti-competitive behaviour. According to the BMA, 'Monitor will also have powers to assist providers in significant difficulty. This will include requiring a provider to appoint a turnaround expert to help them avoid failure, and appointing a continuity administrator to take control of a provider's affairs when it is deemed clinically or financially unsustainable'.

Now let's take a closer look at who is on the **board** of Monitor:[15]

Dr David Bennett (chief executive), ex senior partner at McKinsey & Co (18 years)

Keith Palmer, ex vice chairman of NM Rothschild merchant bank

Sigurd Reinton, director of NATS Holdings (public-private partnership of national air traffic control) and ex director (senior partner) at McKinsey

Heather Lawrence, non-executive director of NMC Healthcare, a FTSE 250 company and member of the Dr Foster Global Comparators Founders Board

Adrian Masters, ex McKinsey, IBM and Price Waterhouse
Stephen Hay, ex KPMG

So Monitor is intended as an independent regulator in the NHS, which will police competition in the NHS and make decisions about hospital trusts, which go bust. Does this really look to you like an independent set of people or, is it likely, in view of their backgrounds, that they will make pro-marketisation and pro-privatisation decisions? This is what you might describe as **regulatory capture**.

While Cameron may pacify us that there will be no switch to an insurance-based model (although he wants to "turn the NHS into a fantastic business"), his new health secretary **Jeremy Hunt** does not agree. It was hard to imagine what could be worse than Andrew Lansley. But his replacement is exactly that—the man **officially on record as saying that the NHS should be privatised.**

Back in 2005, Hunt co-authored with others, including Michael Gove, Tory MEP Daniel 'the NHS is a 60-year-old mistake', Hanaan and Greg Clark, a book called *Direct Democracy* in which they called for the NHS to be dismantled.[16] It's touching to think that a few years ago, in freezing winter, a then unknown MP by the name of Jeremy Hunt joined constituents for a candlelit vigil outside Parliament to highlight that his local hospital—the Royal Surrey in Guildford—was threatened with closure. Even the leader of his party, an apple-cheeked, smooth-faced, young David Cameron, brow as yet unfurrowed by the ordeals of being PM, dropped by to lend his support.[17] One might be forgiven for thinking that this is a classic case of the corrupting effect of power. In fact, this rank hypocrisy is quite prevalent with the same MPs, who voted in favour of the Health & Social Care Act, protesting against hospital cuts and closures in their own constituencies. MPs are still spooked by the 'Kidderminster effect' after Dr Richard Taylor, running as an independent to reinstate the local A&E, won this seat in 2001 with a majority of 18,000 and was even re-elected in 2005.

The Act effectively paves the way for the piecemeal privatisation and break-up of the NHS. Now that the starting gun has been fired, the race to the bottom has officially begun. In October 2012, £262 million of NHS services (mainly community services) were drawing bids from 37 private companies. This was described as the **'biggest act of privatisation ever seen in the NHS'**.[18] In 2013, the Coalition planned to force a further £750 million of services to be opened up to competitive bids. 105 private firms were approved for AQP status. *The Guardian* highlighted some of the winners in this wave of privatisation:

InHealth have been authorised to start operating in 95 places. InHealth earns about £80 million a year from the NHS but plans services at 100 extra locations.

Care UK plans to increase the £190 million a year it earns from NHS patients through 35 new contracts.

Specsavers has won adult hearing contracts in at least 33 places.

Virgin Care has been awarded AQP status in 10 areas for which it applied. It plans to offer dermatology, ophthalmology, ultrasound, podiatry, back and neck pain services and fracture clinics.

BMI Healthcare has begun winning contracts to provide MRI and ultrasound scans.

Plasma Resources UK, which turns plasma into blood products, has been privatised and sold to US private equity company Bain and Company; literally a case of Dracula in charge of the blood bank![19]

Unsurprisingly, the *Financial Times* reported that private sector companies are engaged in an 'arms race' to win NHS contracts.[20] An estimated £2.6 billion worth of contracts have been awarded to profit-driven companies, such as Bupa, Virgin Care and Care UK since the Act came into effect in April 2013. These companies have won 131 contracts so far, or two out of three of the 195 contracts awarded, which represents about half the value of the deals. In the latest wave of privatisation, **Circle** has been the biggest winner with two contracts worth nearly £300 million. **Bupa** has won a contract worth £235 million for musculoskeletal services. At this rate, private firms could earn **£9.2 billion** as a result of these reforms.[21]

Analysis by the Institute of Fiscal Studies and the Nuffield Trust think-tank showed that the slice of the NHS budget going to non-NHS providers (private and voluntary sector) rose from £5.6 billion in 2006-07 to an estimated £8.7 billion in 2011-12 and has now topped £10 billion for the first time.[22] A **£1 billion contract** (later reduced to £800 million) for community health services in Cambridgeshire, which attracted bids from Virgin, Circle and Serco was eventually awarded to an NHS consortium.[23] The contract trumped the value of similar arrangements made with Serco and Virgin to run services in Suffolk (£140 million) and Surrey (£500 million). However, this is not the only contract of this magnitude. Whole service areas are now being offered up. In 2014, a **10-year contract for cancer services** and end of life care in Staffordshire across four CCGs—together worth £1.2 billion—was tendered.[24]

8 reasons why privatisation matters...

- NHS marketisation experiences demonstrate that markets do not work well in healthcare.
- This is further demonstrated by market-based healthcare systems internationally.
- Private providers cut costs (and therefore quality)—by cutting wages (not bound by national wage structures) and staff.
- Private providers are accountable only to shareholder profits cf. public ownership.
- Tendering will lead to fragmentation as opposed to integrated care.
- The bidding process itself is hugely flawed and inefficient.
- Commercial confidentiality allows companies to hide behind a firewall of secrecy despite the public interest at stake.
- Ultimately, it means going down the road of universal private health insurance.

Section 75 is the key part of the Act. The Section 75 regulations pertain to the application of competition within the NHS. However, they caused a furore because they were latched on after the Act had been passed by Parliament. Keep Our NHS Public prepared a parliamentary briefing for MPs likely to be bamboozled by the chicanery of corporate law, having sought legal opinion from David Lock QC. This briefing surmised that the Section 75 regulations close down the current option of an **in-house commissioning process**, even if local people wish it. This option was taken in a number of cases, including *since* the passage of the Act. Ministers confirmed that such arrangements were legal and would not give rise to challenge under **EU procurement law**: 'The regulations sweep all existing arrangements between NHS bodies, and just about all commissioning done by the CCGs, into a market framework—and thus into the remit of **EU competition law**. Once this is triggered, private providers gain rights which make halting their encroachment financially—and thus politically—virtually impossible'.[25]

Confused yet? Well let's think of an example. If your local CCG is deciding who will provide physiotherapy services, it may feel that the local hospital is doing a good job and should therefore continue. Instead, EU competition law will be applied to the tendering of all NHS contracts regardless of whether CCGs see fit or not, with the regulator Monitor having the power to enforce this. This means that **CCGs will be forced to tender out contracts for fear of litigation.**[26] In fact, millions of pounds are already being wasted on legal fees in these tenders.[27] Labour uncovered that **the legal fees to comply with one clause of the Act cost CCGs £77 million a year.**[28]

This gives the lie to the government's claims that clinicians will be in control of decision-making. Of course, **the usual false assurances** were given...

Andrew Lansley: 'There is absolutely nothing in the Bill that promotes or permits the transfer of NHS activities to the private sector'. (13/3/12)

Andrew Lansley's letter to CCGs: 'I know many of you have read that you will be forced to fragment services, or put them out to tender. This is absolutely not the case. It is a fundamental principle of the Bill that you as commissioners, not the Secretary of State and not regulators—should decide when and how competition should be used to serve your patients interests'. (12/2/12)

Simon Burns MP: '...[I]t will be for commissioners to decide which services to tender... [T]o avoid any doubt—it is not the Government's intention that under clause 67 [now 75] that regulations would impose compulsory competitive tendering requirements on commissioners, or for Monitor to have powers to impose such requirements'. (12/7/11)

Lord Howe: 'Clinicians will be free to commission services in the way they consider best. We intend to make it clear that commissioners will have a full range of options and that they will be under no legal obligation to create new markets...'. (6/3/12)

So how does this work in practice? Well the tendering of the NHS Direct telephone service is a good example. It has been 'broken up among 46 bidders for local 111 services, paid only 30% of the old cost per call' leading to contracts going bust whilst under-qualified operators (relying on simplistic algorithms) divert patients inappropriately to A&E.[29] Welcome to the wonderful world of markets!

Had enough yet? Well it only gets worse. Cost is the main consideration for CCGs in the tendering process both due to limited budgets and an obligation to seek value for taxpayer money. Larger companies tend to significantly under-cut on their bids. This strategy is known as a loss leader and is employed because they can afford to take a hit up front and recoup losses in future. However, as one CCG head confided to me, healthcare is not toilet paper. Lower cost simply means lower quality. As the journalist Polly Toynbee puts it, 'more for less' is Toryspeak for less and private. **Serco underbid the NHS trust's best price by**

£10 million on their £140 million contract for community health services in Suffolk. **The result has been staff lay-offs and repeated concerns over poor performance.** Serco is now planning to pull out of clinical services in the NHS and will focus on non-clinical services.

Furthermore, the bidding process is rigged in favour of these larger companies. The simple reason being that a multinational has the resources needed for the complex and costly bidding process, whilst smaller organisations—often public or voluntary sector—do not. **The abandoned competition to run George Eliot hospital cost £1.78 million** with £771,000 going to management consultancies.[30] The tender for the massive Cambridgeshire contract for community services will cost £800,000.[31] I have seen first-hand the time, money and effort poured into bidding for a local GP surgery. All of this would be better used for the benefit of patient care.

The knock-on effect is that smaller competitors, such as charities and co-ops, are edged out, with the result that a cartel develops. This phenomenon can be seen in outsourcing across various sectors. In other words, public sector monopolies—one of the supposed motives for privatisation—are merely replaced by private sector oligopolies.

As for the idea of empowering doctors, only a small number will be on the boards of CCGs. Some of these doctors are entrepreneurial types. Hence why **426 (36%) of the 1,179 GPs in executive positions have a financial interest in a for-profit private provider** beyond their own general practice—a provider from which their CCG could potentially commission services, according to the *British Medical Journal*.[32]

Commissioning Support Units—set up to advise CCGs on how to spend most of the NHS budget—**will be spun-off and privatised.**[33] The usual suspects, including Serco, UnitedHealth and McKinsey will likely bid to take them over. So these multinational companies (rather than clinicians) will advise CCGs on how to purchase services from the same private companies. It's a small world!

Even the American defence giant and international arms company **Lockheed Martin** is considering bidding and attended an NHS England meeting.[34] *The Guardian* has revealed the existence of a **Commissioning Support Industry Group (CSIG)** comprising UnitedHealth, McKinsey, KPMG, Capita, EY and PWC jockeying for commissioning contracts. CSIG receives regular briefings from senior NHS managers. UnitedHealth chairs the group and one of their lobbyists Dr Chris Exeter (previously worked 'on non-health matters for Low Associates, a lobbying firm run by Sally Low, wife of... Andrew Lansley') helps to coordinate meetings.[35]

Foundation Trusts are now allowed to earn 49% of their income from treating private patients. This was previously capped at about 2%. Hospitals are thus preparing to ramp up private patient work to increase incomes in the constraints of the current financial climate. Great Ormond Street Hospital anticipated an extra £11 million from treating private patients in 2013 compared with 2010—that's a 34% increase. Imperial College Healthcare was expecting an extra £9 million over the same period—a 42% rise. Royal Marsden was expecting an extra 28% increase on 2010 revenues, equating to about £12.7 million.Several other trusts, including University College, Royal Brompton, Moorfields, Papworth, Royal Surrey County and Chelsea and Westminster hospitals have all experienced soaring private patient incomes since the passage of the Act.

Across England, there has been **a 10% increase in revenues from private patients compared with 2010.** Out of 146 Foundation Trusts, 40 plan to open private patient units.[36,37] Overt privatisation of hospitals—as with Circle taking over Hinchingbrooke hospital—is politically toxic. So instead we get covert privatisation.

We have already been given a taste of this new NHS with the

arrival on our shores of **Hospital Corporation of America (HCA)—the world's largest private healthcare company**. HCA, co-owned by **Bain Capital**, whose profits helped fund **Mitt Romney's** presidential campaign, is looking to expand further into the NHS. HCA already caters for around half of all private patients in London. NHS England has come under fire after switching gamma knife contracts from the NHS to services run by HCA and Bupa.

Interestingly, private healthcare does not seem to operate along the lines of the idealised Adam Smith universe that neoliberals envisage. The Competition Commission's report— 'Private healthcare in central London: horizontal competitive constraints'—focused on the lack of competition and overcharging in the private healthcare market. The Centre for Health and the Public Interest (CHPI) published a report in 2013 warning that 'greater use of for-profit providers as a result of the Health Act is likely to substantially increase the amount of healthcare fraud in the NHS'. This would specifically be through overcharging to maximise shareholder returns. *The Independent* points out that **'HCA had to pay more than $1.7bn in fraud settlements in the US in 2003 after admitting 14 felonies'.** [38]

According to a *New York Times* investigation, the factors behind HCA's rapid growth included more revenue from insurance companies, patients and Medicare through 'much more aggressive billing' and reducing expenses.

Step Eight:
Plot Against the NHS

Now if I told you that we have not even got to the most remarkable part of this story then you'd probably think I was lying. But you'd be wrong. Pretty much everything in this narrative was hatched in **a series of think-tank documents from the 1980s**—that something can be so faithfully executed over 25 years is a testament to Machiavellianism.

Dr Lucy Reynolds and Professor Martin McKee have charted this journey:

'[In the late 1980s]... a conference attended by Conservative politicians, NHS senior managers and think-tank advisors set out a seven-step plan to alter the NHS... In 1988, the pro-market Centre for Policy Studies (CPS) published a series of short studies exploring this agenda... One study was published as a pamphlet entitled **"Britain's biggest enterprise" by Conservative MPs Oliver Letwin and John Redwood'.**[1]

Here is an excerpt from 'Britain's biggest enterprise':

'Might it not, rather, be possible to work slowly from the present system towards a national insurance scheme? One could begin for example, with the establishment of the NHS as an independent trust, with increased joint ventures between the NHS and the private sector; move on next to the use of "credits" to meet standard charges set by central NHS funding administration for independently managed hospitals or districts; and only at the last stage create a national health scheme separate from the tax system'.[2]

It is worth noting that, around this time, Letwin and Redwood headed NM Rothschild bank's international privatisation unit and that Letwin had published a book called *Privatising the World* with a foreword by Redwood. (Just in case you're in any doubt as to the intentions of this dastardly duo and the Tories more generally towards the NHS, as some media commentators seem to be.)

Oliver **Letwin** has a Nostradamus-like tendency (or perhaps these are simply self-fulfilling prophecies when you are pulling the strings). *The Independent* reported in 2004 that Letwin told a private meeting the **NHS will not exist within 5 years of a Conservative government**. Two weeks previously, Letwin's plans for massive cuts to public spending were also leaked.[3] It is worth highlighting that this was long before any hint of a financial crisis. Both reports were, of course, strenuously denied!

In 1988, Madsen Pirie co-authored a paper called 'The Health of Nations' for the Adam Smith Institute.[4] This anticipated future reforms from the internal market, public-private partnerships, foundation trusts and competitive tendering through to personal health budgets.

The Health & Social Care Act itself has been gestating for years and can be directly traced back to a speech Lansley made in 2005. The speech drew on his formative experiences as a civil servant involved in utility privatisations. **Lansley had been private secretary to Norman Tebbit when Tebbit was privatising BT**. As Nicholas Timmins documents in *Never Again: The Story of the Health & Social Care Act*, the full details emerged in 2007 in a white paper entitled 'NHS Autonomy and Accountability'. Right there, in the rubric, was the proposal for the private sector to bid for NHS work with no cap on the share they might secure. The other keynote ideas were already in place too—an NHS commissioning board with GPs in the driving seat, a new economic regulator to promote competition and all hospitals to become foundation trusts.[5]

In light of all this, the recent admission by senior Tories on the front page of *The Times* that the NHS reforms were their biggest mistake has to be seen as a cynical election ploy![6] This article claimed that David Cameron did not understand the reforms. Either that or he is complicit in knowingly destroying our NHS. Guilty or incompetent? Whichever it is, he does not come out of this well. This may help to explain how he had the nerve in his Conference speech in 2014 to state that he cares deeply about the NHS because it looked after his disabled son Ivan.

Step Nine:
Brew the Perfect Storm

This is just the beginning. The NHS is being transformed into an umbrella for private provider purchasing, reduced to an insignia with enormous brand recognition. It's all very well for Cameron to reassure us that the NHS remains free at the point of delivery (for the time being) funded by general taxation. But this is of little solace when the cost to the taxpayer has become exorbitant, whilst the private sector is enriched beyond measure.

Never let a crisis go to waste so they say. McKinsey heeded this advice following the financial crisis, and produced a report 'Achieving World Class Productivity in the NHS 2009/10-2013/14: Detailing the Size of the Opportunity'. This recommended shedding up to 10% of staff i.e. 135,000 people and led to the efficiency savings dubbed the Nicholson challenge. Nicholson's intolerant response to those opposing NHS reforms was: 'There are people in the service who essentially hate all this [i.e. Lansley's plans]. My view is that they should go'.

The looming NHS performance crisis is already unfolding, with projected NHS efficiency savings of £15-20 billion up to 2015. *The Telegraph* reports that as many as one in five hospitals are facing closures of some kind, A&Es and maternity wards are being shut down and thousands of NHS staff have been sacked, with waiting lists inevitably going up.[1] The *Daily Mail* even launched its own Save Our Hospitals campaign.

The dire situation in nursing exemplifies the chaos. Whilst the government cuts nurse training places, hospitals are forced to hire more expensive agency nurses, often from abroad. Likewise, numbers of district and community nurses are plunging, with district nurses down from 12,500 in 2003 to 7,500 presently.[2]

All of which highlights the hypocrisy at the heart of the NHS reforms. Cameron and Hunt talk about patient choice, improving standards and empowering healthcare professionals. Yet their policies enact the opposite through cuts, closures, sacking staff and privatisation. They may trumpet the slogan 'No decision about me without me' but what about the decision to privatise the NHS? I do not recall this decision being made with our consent.

The unravelling or how it will play out...

1) PFI debts will be a major factor in NHS trusts allowed to 'go bust'.

2) Efficiency savings—or cuts—will be extended for years to come. This is a common fate of public sector organisations in which they are starved of cash and deliberately run into the ground. At which point, privatisation is conjured up as the unavoidable panacea.

3) Compulsory competitive tendering of all contracts to Any Qualified Provider leads to cherry-picking. This means that high-volume, low-risk healthcare is picked off by private firms leading to unbundling of services and therefore a smaller pot of money to provide comprehensive healthcare, which in turn leads to increased rationing.

Think of your local hospital. This hospital is paid for the treatments and services it provides. It makes money from straightforward procedures like cataracts or hip and knee replacements. This money is then used to pay for expensive and risky healthcare like emergency medicine and intensive care. However, when the former has been cherry-picked by companies like Virgin and Serco then this money is permanently siphoned off out of the system leaving less to pay for the latter. To give one example, Circle had taken 30% of the market share for hip, ankle and knee operations in the Bath area from 2010-11.[3] This, in turn, destabilises local health economies. So when David Cameron stands at the dispatch box and states that it does not matter who provides healthcare as long as it is free at the point of delivery then this is a big, fat lie. And he knows it.

Furthermore, competitive tendering leads to fragmentation rather than integrated care—the buzzword of policy wonks.[4] Take the diabetic care pathway, which requires complex coordinated management—foot and eye care, diet and lifestyle education, optimising of blood sugar control and medication, monitoring of other risk factors like blood pressure and cholesterol. If this is fragmented amongst different providers (often not communicating with each other) then the quality of care deteriorates. Ideally this care should all be carried out by one provider. It makes much more sense to have collaboration rather than competition in healthcare.

Once you combine all of the above factors then you have a perfect storm in which the NHS withers away. Rationing of care is already accelerating. A *British Medical Journal* survey showed that **one in seven CCGs have brought in new restrictions over what treatment people can get**, including those for recurrent migraines, new barriers to joint replacement and cataract operations.[5] In some areas, only one cataract is removed. Apparently one eye is enough! **A CCG in Devon has recently announced that obese patients and smokers will be denied all routine surgery, shoulder surgery will be restricted for all patients and hearing aids will be available for only one ear not two.**[6] In fact, these rationing and funding decisions can then be ascribed to doctors on CCGs rather than blamed on the government.

Rationing will become more widespread until we have a two-tier system in which the haves will be forced to take out private insurance and the have-nots will be looked after by a third-class health service. This is how you privatise the NHS by stealth.

PFI claimed its first scalp during the summer of 2012. **South London Healthcare Trust (SLHT) became the first NHS trust to go bust** after debts started accumulating at a rate of £1.3 million per week.[7] In fact, there are **two PFI hospitals in SLHT with a combined projected cost of £2 billion**—the Queen Elizabeth in Woolwich and the Princess Royal in Bromley, which will cost the NHS £1.2 billion alone, more than 10 times what they are worth.[8] SLHT has the dubious honour of being the first trust to enter the Unsustainable Providers Regime. It was then announced that neighbouring Lewisham's A&E and maternity services would be sacrificed—presumably in order to keep servicing PFI repayments—despite Lewisham being a solvent, well-managed stand-alone trust. Based on precedents, the downgrading of emergency and acute care services is often the precursor to shutting down the whole hospital.

The Trust Special Administrator did not count on the Save Lewisham Hospital campaign. The turnout was estimated at 25,000 at its second demonstration. To think there were only a handful of people at the first organising meeting. The campaign, aided by 38 Degrees, took Jeremy Hunt to the High Court and won. **A judicial review ruled that government plans were illegal.**[9] This sets an important legal precedent that when PFI trusts are bankrupt, they should not be restructured at the expense of their neighbours. Ever the bad losers, the Tories tried to change the law, handing special administrators enhanced powers for restructuring hospital trusts so that they will be unencumbered in future.[10]

The restructuring plans for SLHT demonstrated that **an NHS trust could be dismantled in as quickly as 18 weeks.** The sobering lesson is that, if a successful hospital like Lewisham is in danger of being downgraded, then no hospital is safe. NHS trusts should not be restructured through no fault of their own—leading to mergers, closures and shrinkage—when neighbouring trusts incur deficits. And as we have seen before, these deficits are often incurred through factors beyond their control like PFI payments indexed higher with each year. SLHT is a test case that can be rolled out across the country. There are now at least 20

NHS trusts, comprising around 60 hospitals, in danger of going bust with PFI debts as a major contributory factor.[11]

COMING SOON TO A HOSPITAL NEAR YOU

NHS North West London has recently made the decision to downgrade four A&Es with plans to virtually close down over 300 beds at Charing Cross and near total closure of in-patient care at the 327-bed Ealing Hospital. This means there will be **no A&E for the boroughs of Hammersmith & Fulham, Ealing and Brent—a population of 750,000, or a city the size of Leeds**. The prospect is of 'almost 1,000 bed cuts by 2015 in North West London, averaging 28 per cent cuts across all eight West London boroughs. This includes drastic cuts by 2015 of around a third of beds in three hospitals set to carry the additional workload when the A&Es are closed—Chelsea & Westminster, West Middlesex and Northwick Park'.[12]

Without investment in local community and GP services, this is surely the recipe for pushing already overstretched resources to breaking point. NHS North West London executives have been forced to admit publicly, 'there are **NO concrete plans to establish alternative, community-based services** to take the place of the axed hospitals'.[13]

Around 55% of the Charing Cross site and 45% of the St Mary's site will be sold off. The sale of NHS land and property is irreversible.[14] At the same time, Imperial College Healthcare Trust plans to double its private patient income. Yet there is money to be made, even when it comes to these closures. McKinsey has been paid more than £3.5 million for this work in North West London as part of the ironically titled 'Shaping a Healthier Future' reconfiguration.[15]

Similar plans for 'reconfiguration' or closure are unfolding in South West London—affecting Kingston, Epsom and St Helier hospitals—and are heading for East London. According to the *Daily Telegraph*, there are 66 implemented/planned A&E and maternity unit closures across the country.[16]

Polly Toynbee summed it up nicely in *The Guardian*: 'Follow the money: **£300m** is being tendered out by Monitor… to pay the administration costs of the "failure regime" for **up to 60 bankrupt trusts over four years**…. The notorious Mid-Staffordshire hospital has **£2.5m to pay McKinsey and Ernst & Young** as registered insolvency practitioners: these are just starter sums, with much more for reconfiguration. The failed South London trust has **£5m for McKinsey and Deloitte**, more to come. McKinsey is the big NHS player likely to get the lion's share, as Mid Yorks, North Yorks, Epsom, St Helier, Morecambe, Barking, Peterborough, the Friarage, Imperial, Barts and scores more head towards the NHS Unsustainable Providers Regime.'[17]

Breaking the allegiance and loyalty of staff is one of the important strategies for attacking a public sector organisation. This is often achieved through policies that demoralise and alienate them. Under the coalition, we have seen reforms to pensions, meaning that staff will effectively have to pay more, retire later and get less. There has been a year-on-year public sector pay freeze despite the independent NHS Pay Review Body recommending a 1% pay rise for all NHS staff in 2014. Jeremy Hunt rejected this recommendation.[18] It is likely that automatic pay rises (linked to length of service in the public sector) and merit awards for excellence will be phased out. New GP and hospital consultant contracts are to be forced upon doctors, which will again mean more work for less money. A new sub-consultant grade will be created, thus reducing the number of senior consultants.

Francis Maude—the former Conservative Party Chairman and current Minister for the Cabinet Office—talks of running more hospitals and even emergency services outside the public sector. He floated the idea of mutual companies owned by employees. Maude also warned that more public sector jobs will be axed with further wage cuts.[19] Other possible models would include joint public-private ventures. As Professor Martin McKee points out, John Lewis is usually cited as the shining example of mutualisation, although the reality is not always so benevolent. The Circle Health model may be more applicable, with employees holding a minority stake whilst the real power lies with hedge funds. Unlike Germany, we do not currently have the legal safeguards to stop private equity buy-outs or corporate takeovers of mutualised hospitals. This is really a thinly-disguised shrinking of the public sector and privatisation by a different name.[20]

This is in keeping with David Cameron's 'Big Society' concept. However, as we have seen, the voluntary sector— charities, co-operatives, mutuals—do not appear to be the main beneficiary. The big society actually means a return to the pre-welfare state days, in other words to a Victorian world in which healthcare and welfare are not the responsibility of the state but of philanthropic organisations and individuals. This is clearly a regressive direction of travel for the country.

Step Ten:
Introduce Universal
Private Health Insurance

Personal health budgets: a Trojan horse

Personal health budgets are exactly what they sound like—a patient can use money directly for purchasing health and other services. For example, they might purchase a block of physiotherapy sessions for £500. Or they might feel that they would better use that money on gym membership. Or buying a bike. Personal health budgets have been used for personal care for many years. Pilots are now being rolled out to 50,000 patients and will be extended nationwide from April 2015.[1] It's all about empowerment, right?

Wrong. They represent the **logical end-point of the journey with the self-paying consumer in a market for healthcare**. The real question is what happens when your personal health budget runs out. Easy, you top it up. Or not so easy if you don't have the money. In other words, they enable insurance for top-ups (co-payments). Hence why insurance companies like WPA and AXA PPP are reportedly enthusiastic. At the same time, Bupa has been busy preparing its own clinical guidelines and creating networks of doctors gearing up for this brave, new world. Personal health budgets undermine the fundamental NHS principle of equity of care. They are a Trojan horse for privatisation.

The publication of the Dalton review in December 2014, commissioned by the government, has looked at whether public or private companies could own and operate chains of hospitals. Case studies for this review included Spain and Germany, where privately-run public hospitals have expanded. Alternatively, this might pave the way for 'new conglomerations of super NHS trusts, some privately managed', which could entice private investors and even buy-outs from private equity groups.[2]

So we will have budget-holding patients under an NHS modelled on state insurance providers like Medicare in the United States, with CCGs acting as insurance pools—able to exclude undesirable patients, buying healthcare from private companies and making funding decisions supported by privatised commissioning support units. Top-up co-payments as well as care pathways and packages would then allow integration of this system with private healthcare insurance giants.

Although ministers, including Prime Minister David Cameron, continue to omit the P word, what is happening on the ground is clearly privatisation according to the **World Health Organisation definition of healthcare privatisation: 'a process in which non-governmental actors become increasingly involved in the financing and/or provision of healthcare services'.**

You see, the privatisation of the NHS affects us all. One bandies around the platitude that you never know when you will need the NHS. But as a fit young person, you don't seriously believe it. Until something happens, as I discovered in 2013 when I ruptured my Achilles tendon playing football—the textbook injury of the dilettante weekend sports-player. I was on crutches for 4 months under the care of the orthopaedic team and then required weekly physiotherapy for several months after. At the same time, my father—a retired Consultant Psychiatrist—was very unwell in hospital, requiring intensive care at one point. We have since both made a good recovery thanks to the NHS. To think that the government allied with the private healthcare sector wants to take the right to healthcare away from each and every one of us—when we are at our most vulnerable—makes my blood boil.

At the time, I was invited to a patient workshop at a large, central London teaching hospital at which one of the consultants spoke of the increasing numbers of patients and how this would be good news if only they were a business. The irony did not pass by unnoticed, as I thought to myself gosh you are a business in all but name. As a foundation trust, they are paid by throughput in a market-based system. They are free to make partnerships with companies and up to half their income can come from private patients.

As for general practice, the abolition of the Minimum Practice Income Guarantee means that more than 100 surgeries, in deprived parts of the country, may have to close. This will be coupled with cuts to GP funding (imposing an average formula across the board), thus not taking into account the extra spending needed for deprived areas. I work in Tower Hamlets, where the life expectancy of our patients is 10-15 years shorter than other parts of London. Some practices will lose hundreds of thousands of pounds a year. Again, the result will be either closure or a massive reduction in what they can offer. It is likely that GP surgeries will be forced to merge, attracting private investment and facilitating takeovers.

GP contracts will likely be converted to APMS (where contracts can be made with companies employing salaried GPs) to comply with competition rules. This means that **all GP contracts would then be tendered and are open to privatisation** and franchising.[3] APMS contracts last 5 years, which will also encourage short-term profiteering rather than long term investment in public health. It will also spell the end of the traditional model of family doctors.

As if we do not already have enough to worry about, there is **the Transatlantic Trade and Investment Partnership (TTIP)**. Linda Kaucher has untangled the subtext of TTIP in an article for Open Democracy.[4] She explains that this EU-US trade agreement, like all 'trade agreements', is effectively an 'irreversible commitment made at the level of international law, i.e. beyond changes at the level of the UK government or the EU'. Financial services is a major force for the **liberalisation** of public services opening them up to transnational investors and thus privatisation. When public services are committed to 'international trade agreements, the liberalisation of those services is then locked in' i.e. irreversible.

TTIP gives transnational corporations rights to:

- Operate without limits on activities, or on the number of transnational corporations that enter the sector.
- Same or better treatment than national companies.
- Rights to sue government in an international jurisdiction if there is any attempt to limit rights or introduce regulation which might limit corporations' expected future profits. These are called **investor-state dispute settlements (ISDS)**.

ISDS allows corporate lawyers to sue governments in secretive, private courts. Other trade agreements have already facilitated countless examples of corporations suing governments over measures taken for the public good. Phillip Morris has sued the Australian government over plain packaging for cigarettes. A Swedish firm is suing the German government over the decision to ban nuclear power. Argentina was sued by international utility firms over freezing energy and water bills and has been forced to shell out over a billion dollars for this and other such claims.[5] In the first 16 years of the North American Free Trade Agreement (NAFTA), Canada, Mexico and the US 'faced 66 such claims costing several hundred million dollars in compensation and legal fees'.

ISDS essentially acts as a deterrent to prevent governments acting against corporate interests. The Labour Party has promised to repeal the Health & Social Care Act but even so, TTIP would still lock in privatisation and might well mean that it would be too costly to renationalise NHS services. Labour have also vowed to exempt the NHS from TTIP but this is not a straightforward matter due to complex legal mechanisms.[6]

In fact, it is possible that the Health & Social Care Act was drawn up with TTIP in mind. Health would then be the first sector to be *harmonised*, meaning that regulations will be aligned between the EU and US. However, regulatory 'harmonisation' with the US will be much broader. Another obvious target for 'harmonisation' is the European public broadcasting model. So the BBC, whose public duty is to inform you of what is in this book, will be next in the line of fire.

The Health & Social Care Act is a centerpiece policy that has to be seen in the context of the wider Conservative project. The Tories are taking a wrecking ball to the state. In two years, the Coalition has set in motion the dismantling of the welfare state on a scale that Thatcher could scarcely have dreamed of. The chutzpah is breath-taking and one is left asking how they manage to get away with it. As the spectre of austerity sweeps through Europe, the social contract is being ripped up. The electro-shock therapy applied to Greece is an experiment that can be implemented elsewhere. After decades of wreaking havoc across the world, **neoliberalism writ large—in the form of privatisation, deregulation and shrinking the state**—has come home to roost.

The NHS was created in the wake of World War II during a time of real austerity and shared suffering in a society based on communal values. As Peter Wilby has pointed out, this 'collectivism came naturally to people who had emerged from a devastating war that required patience, stoicism and personal sacrifice for the common good'. On the first day of the NHS, some doctors barricaded themselves in their offices anticipating a stampede. Instead patients formed an orderly queue.[7]

After 30 years of neoliberalism, we have a fragmented, atomised society of hyper-individualism. In other words, the collective ethos of the public sector comes into collision with the consumerist culture of instant gratification in which the concept of waiting is intolerable. As Wilby sums it up, 'Public services, free at the point of use, cannot work as goods and services offered through the private sector market do. They provide to all at low public cost what would otherwise be available only to some at high private cost... Nobody expects a bus to turn up at a time of their choosing as a taxi would'.

Are the NHS and the welfare state compatible with this new world? That's the question millions of people—particularly young people—are going to have to figure out for themselves. Bevan's vision was to ensure that healthcare was never again a commodity. Sadly we are regressing back to that pre-NHS world, where healthcare is distributed according to ability to pay rather than need. **The British public has not been consulted on this momentous decision that arguably affects each of us more than anything in our lives. These government policies, which will harm the health of an entire nation, carried out without the consent of the people, are nothing less than an act of betrayal.**

As Martin Luther King once said, **'Of all the forms of inequality, injustice in health care is the most shocking and inhumane'.**

Resistance is NOT futile. This is a call to arms.

One only has to look at the devolved countries to see the NHS in its original remit—as a publicly funded, publicly provided and publicly accountable service. Scotland has turned its back on PFI and abolished the internal market after devolution. Scottish Futures Trust, owned by the government, has been set up to finance infrastructure projects.[8]

The survival of the NHS is imperilled and it is on the verge of extinction. It's up to all of us.

What can you do?

Retain our NHS as a publicly provided, publicly funded and publicly accountable service by supporting the **Campaign for an NHS Reinstatement Bill:**

http://www.nhsbill2015.org.

Join/follow **National Health Action Party**: www.nhap.org.

Exert pressure on the **Labour Party.**

Write to your local **MP.**

If you are a doctor then be active in your **BMA** local division and consider joining the **MPU**

Unite have launched an NHS campaign.

Arrange a local meeting with **38 Degrees** for concerned people in your area.

Attend local **Keep Our NHS Public** meetings: www.keepournhspublic.com.

When Aneurin Bevan was sceptically asked how long the NHS would survive, he replied, '**As long as there are folk left with the faith to fight for it'.**

The biggest weapon in this fight will be you—patients and the public. Thousands of people are using GP surgeries and hospitals every day. If we can get the word out to them of what is happening, then the momentum of a national campaign to save the NHS will be unstoppable.

Labour MP Clive Efford's NHS (amended duties and powers) Bill could be a start. This private member's bill aims to repeal some of the worst elements of the Health & Social Care Act (particularly Section 75 and enforced competitive tendering), reintroduce the private patient income cap, exempt the NHS from TTIP and restore the health secretary's responsibility for the NHS.[9] However, some critics feel it does not go far enough and will not halt the privatisation programme.

The historic events of 2011 are testimony to what people power can achieve. When people united in solidarity and spoke truth to power then the paper tigers, whether media moguls or Middle East dictators, crumbled and were scattered to the wind. May you live in interesting times as they say.

We started with a few questions about the NHS. I have tried to answer them. But now it's my turn. I have one question for David Cameron:

WHO GAVE YOU PERMISSION TO BREAK UP OUR NHS AND SELL IT OFF?

Reading list

Books

NHS SOS – Jacky Davis and Raymond Tallis (eds.), Oneworld, 2013

The Plot Against the NHS – Colin Leys and Stewart Player, The Merlin Press, 2011

NHS Plc – Allyson Pollock, Verso, 2005

Papers

Opening the oyster: the 2010–11 NHS reforms in England – RCP Clinical Medicine 2012 Vol 12, No2:128-32 Lucy Reynolds & Martin McKee

Health and Social Care Bill 2011: a legal basis for charging and providing fewer health services to people in England – *British Medical Journal* 17/3/12 Allyson Pollock, David Price, Peter Roderick

Further resources

www.guardian.co.uk/society/series/nhs-plc

www.defendlondonsnhs.wordpress.com

References

Introduction

1. Preface, *The Plot Against the NHS* by Colin Leys and Stewart Player. The Merlin Press – 2011.
2. The Ultimate Indignity of the A&E Closures, *Daily Mail*, 23/11/13.
3. Ken Clarke quote from 'Never Again? The story of the health and social care act' by Nicholas Timmins.

Chapter 1

1. Karen Bloor et al., "NHS Management and Administration Staffing and Expenditure in a National and International Context", March 2005 as referenced in Health Committee Fourth report on Commissioning 18/3/10.
2. The billions of wasted NHS cash no-one wants to mention – Caroline Molloy Open Democracy 10/10/14.

Chapter 2

1. *The Plot against the NHS*, Chapter 1 on Tim Evans and the concordat.
2. *The Plot Against the NHS*, Chapter 1 on ISTCs.
3. BMA pamphlet Look After Our NHS – February 2010 – original source Department of Health & Parliament Health Select Committee 2007-8.
4. 'NHS privatisation keeps on failing patients', *The Guardian* 15/8/14.
5. 'PFI contracts: the full list', *Guardian* datablog (Source HM Treasury) 5/7/12.
6. 'Must we sack teachers to pay for £320 plug sockets', *Daily Telegraph* 25/1/11.
7. 'Private Finance Initiative: hospitals will bring taxpayers 60 years of pain', *Daily Telegraph* 24/1/11.

8. 'Financial crunch tips NHS towards £1bn deficit', *The Guardian* 16/9/14.

9. Health & Social Care Information Centre for numbers and salaries.

10. BMA 'How much does it cost to train a doctor in the United Kingdom?' and 'The cost of surgical training' by the Association of Surgeons in Training & Royal College of Surgeons in England.

11. Papworth Hospital NHS Trust Website.

12. NHS: what we give and what we get, *BBC News* 11/4/06.

13. 'Must we sack teachers to pay for £320 plug sockets', *Daily Telegraph* 25/1/11.

14. PFI contracts: the full list, *Guardian* datablog (Source HM Treasury) 5/7/12.

15. Barts Health interest rates taken from Sir Richard Sykes Chairman of Imperial College NHS Trust as quoted in 'Charing Cross Sell-Off vital to avoid disastrous PFI deal' by Ross Lydall 26/9/14.

16. 'Private Finance Initiative: hospitals will bring taxpayers 60 years of pain', *Daily Telegraph* 24/1/11.

17. Innisfree website.

18. How PFI is crippling the NHS, *The Guardian* 29/6/12.

19. 'PFI schemes will cost every household nearly £400 next year', *Telegraph* 28/4/11.

20. New Economics Foundation Mythbusters, 'The private sector is more efficient than the public sector' April 2013.

21. Report: New PFI initiative will saddle NHS trusts with worse debts than before, *The Independent* 26/11/14.

Chapter 3

1. See *The Plot Against the NHS* for more on GP contracts, outsourcing of OOH care, APMS contracts, integrated care and foundation trusts.

2. 'Serco investigated over claims of "unsafe" out of hours GP

service', *The Guardian* 25/5/12.

3. 'Services provider established by outsourcing giant Serco overcharged NHS by millions', *The Independent* 27/8/14.

4. 'Former Harmoni clinician warns of 'dangerous' pressure on appointments', *The Guardian* 18/12/12.

5. See *The Plot Against the NHS*, Chapter 3 for more on OOH outsourcing.

6. 'The NHS is on the brink: can it survive till May 2015?', *The Guardian* 9/5/14.

7. Do we have too many hospitals?, *British Medical Journal* 13/2/14 2014;348:g1374 John Appleby.

8. See *The Plot Against the NHS*, Chapter 2 on payment by results.

9. 'The billions of wasted NHS cash no-one wants to mention', Caroline Molloy, Open Democracy 10/10/14.

10. Planning for closure: the role of special administrators in reducing NHS hospital services in England – British Medical Journal 2013;347:f7322 13/12/13.

Chapter 4

1. See *The Plot Against the NHS* for more on the revolving door.

2. 'Spending breakdown reveals how NHS England cash flowed to private firms', *The Guardian* 27/11/14.

3. Behind closed doors: how much power does McKinsey wield – British Medical Journal 2008; 337:a2673 12/5/12.

4. 'Health trusts spend £300m on private consultants', *The Guardian* 20/8/10.

5. 'NHS spending on management consultants doubles under the Coalition', *Telegraph* 9/12/14.

6. 'Accenture escapes £1bn penalty for NHS walk-out', *The Register* 29/9/06, originally published on Kablenet.

7. Nick Seddon material from 'This can't go on' by Andrew Robertson of Social Investigations for Open Democracy 13/5/13.

8. 'Selling-Off NHS for profit', *Daily Mirror* 17/11/14 and 'NHS Privatisation: Compilation of financial & vested interests',

Social Investigations Blog 18/2/12.

9. 'Companies with links to Tories 'have won £1.5bn worth of NHS contracts', *The Guardian* 3/10/14.

Chapter 5

1. 'Serco: the company that is running Britain', *The Guardian* 29/7/13.
2. 'Lockheed and the Future of Warfare', *New York Times* 28/11/04.
3. See *The Plot Against the NHS* on UnitedHealth & Netcare.
4. Fortune website.
5. 'UnitedHealth Sues Insurance Commissioner', *USA Today* 11/7/14.
6. 'Calls for greater disclosure on NHS chiefs' meetings with private US health insurer', *The Guardian* 30/8/14.
7. 'The firm that hijacked the NHS', *Mail on Sunday* 12/2/12.

Chapter 6

1. Department of Health factsheets 'Overview of the Health & Social Care Act' 30/4/12.
2. Can we afford the NHS in future? British Medical Journal 2011;343:d4321 12/7/11 John Appleby.
3. 'Why the health service needs surgery by Andrew Lansley', *Telegraph* 1/6/11.
4. 'Financial crisis is inevitable in the NHS', *British Medical Journal News* 10/5/14.
5. Rises in healthcare spending: where will it end? British Medical Journal 2012;345:e7127 1/11/12 John Appleby.
6. Why the US healthcare system is failing, and what might rescue it – British Medical Journal 2012;344:e3052 9/5/12.
7. The NHS belongs to the people: a call to action, NHS England 11/7/13.
8. 'New Tory-appointed NHS boss admits: "I don't use the NHS"', *Daily Mirror* 30/10/11.

9. A Guide to the Reforms, Keep Our NHS Public.

10. 'DH to hand over billions of pounds underspend to Treasury', *Pulse Magazine* 21/8/13.

11. 'A Decade of Austerity?', Nuffield Trust 3/12/12.

12. A productivity challenge too far? – British Medical Journal 2012;344:e2416 19/6/12 John Appleby.

13. NHS finances: the tanker en route for the iceberg – British Medical Journal Editorials 10/5/14.

14. See *The Plot Against the NHS*.

15. 'NHS is the world's best healthcare system', *The Guardian* 17/6/14.

16. 2011 Commonwealth Fund report and Mirror, Mirror on the Wall, 2014 Update: How the U.S. Health Care System Compares Internationally.

17. 'Coalition health bill will undermine NHS, says OECD thinktank', *The Guardian* 23/11/11.

18. 'London NHS hospital trust Barts Health losing £2m a week', *The Guardian* 17/7/13.

19. 'A quarter of walk-in centres have been closed since 2010', *The Guardian* 11/11/13.

20. 'Why A&E departments are fighting for their life', *The Guardian* 14/1/14.

21. 'NHS trusts are enmeshed in private provision - as buyers and suppliers', *The Guardian* 18/12/12.

22. 'Hospitals under pressure as "bedblocking" hits record levels', *The Guardian* 28/11/14.

23. 'NHS care at home for elderly and disabled quietly slashed by a third', *Daily Telegraph* 14/1/14.

24. A Guide to the Reforms, Keep Our NHS Public.

25. Does poor health justify NHS reform? – British Medical Journal 2011;342:d566 28/1/11 John Appleby.

26. 'Better data means better care in the NHS', *The Guardian* 2/12/12.

27. 'British Social Attitudes Survey - how what we think and

who thinks it has changed', *The Guardian* 17/9/12.

28. Britons are more proud of their history, NHS and army than the Royal Family, Ipsos Mori 21/3/12.

29. 'Coalition health bill will undermine NHS, says OECD thinktank', *The Guardian* 23/11/11.

Chapter 7

1. 'David Cameron is accused of a 'sham listening exercise' on NHS reform after links to lobbyist are revealed', *The Guardian* 25/11/12.

2. *Never Again: The Story of the Health & Social Care Act*, Nicholas Timmins.

3. Equity and Excellence: Liberating the NHS White Paper - 12/7/10.

4. 'It is the only change management system you can actually see from space – it is that large', Sir David Nicholson, former NHS chief executive.

5. 'David Cameron is accused of a 'sham listening exercise' on NHS reform after links to lobbyist are revealed', *The Guardian* 25/11/12.

6. 'This can't go on', Andrew Robertson of Social Investigations for Open Democracy 13/5/13.

7. 'The day they signed the death warrant for the NHS', *Daily Telegraph* 25/7/11.

8. 'It's already happened', James Meek, London Review of Books 22/9/11.

9. Cameron: The First Cut, Anthony Seldon, Institute for Public Policy Research 30/9/14.

10. 'It's already happened', James Meek, London Review of Books 22/9/11.

11. Opportunities Post Global Healthcare reforms, Apax Partners October 2010.

12. *Never Again: The Story of the Health & Social Care Act*, Nicholas Timmins.

13. What we know so far... the Health & Social Care Act 2012 at a glance - British Medical Association April 2012.

14. Health and Social Care Bill 2011: a legal basis for charging and providing fewer health services to people in England BMJ 2012;344:e1729, Allyson Pollock, David Price and Peter Roderick 8/3/12.

15. Monitor board from www.gov.uk website.

16. 'Key Tory MPs backed call to dismantle NHS', *The Observer* 16/8/09.

17. 'You must stop A&E cuts: Powerful lobby of 140 top doctors sign damning letter to PM', *Daily Mail* 7/10/12.

18. 'NHS being "atomised" by expansion of private sector's role, say doctors', *The Guardian* 6/1/13.

19. 'Bain Capital buys majority stake in Plasma Resources UK', *The Guardian* 18/7/13.

20. '"Arms race"' over £5bn in NHS work', *Financial Times* 29/7/13 and '£5.8bn of NHS work being advertised to private sector', *Financial Times* 29/7/14.

21. 'Private firms on course to net £9bn of NHS contracts', *The Guardian* 18/7/14.

22. 'Rise in bailouts as more hospitals overspend on budgets', *The Guardian* 22/7/14.

23. 'NHS privatisation fears deepen over £1bn deal', *The Guardian* 26/7/13.

24. 'NHS cancer care could switch to private contracts in £700m plans', *The Guardian* 2/7/14.

25. Keep Our NHS Public Parliamentary Briefing 21/2/13.

26. 'The NHS at 65: chaos, queues and mounting costs', *The Guardian* 5/7/13.

27. A healthy market? Lack of transparency raises doubts about NHS commissioning – British Medical Journal 2013;347:f 7115 4/12/13.

28. 'The billions of wasted NHS cash no-one wants to mention', Caroline Molloy, Open Democracy 10/10/14.

29. 'The NHS at 65: chaos, queues and mounting costs', *The Guardian* 5/7/13.

30. NHS spent £1.8m on abandoned George Eliot competition, Health Service Journal 7/10/14.

31. 'The billions of wasted NHS cash no-one wants to mention', Caroline Molloy, Open Democracy 10/10/14.

32. More than a third of GPs on commissioning groups have conflicts of interest – British Medical Journal 14/3/13 2013;346:f1569.

33. 'NHS approaches equity groups for services takeover', *Financial Times* 3/11/13.

34. 'International arms firm Lockheed Martin in the frame for £1bn NHS contract', *The Independent* 19/11/14.

35. 'Calls for greater disclosure on NHS chiefs' meetings with private US health insurer', *The Guardian* 30/8/14.

36. 'Private patient income soars at NHS trusts', *The Guardian* 19/8/14.

37. 'NHS trusts chasing private patients at expense of waiting lists, warns Labour,' *Observer* 16/11/14.

38. 'World's largest private healthcare company HCA plans expansion into NHS', *The Independent* 14/6/13.

Chapter 8

1. Opening the Oyster: the 2010-11 NHS reforms in England - RCP Clinical Medicine 2012 Vol 12, No2:128-32 Lucy Reynolds & Martin McKee.

2. Britain's biggest enterprise, Oliver Letwin and John Redwood for the Centre for Policy Studies 1988.

3. 'Letwin: "NHS will not exist under Tories"', *The Independent* 6/6/04.

4. 'The Health of Nations', Madsen Pirie for the Adam Smith Institute 1988.

5. *Never Again: The Story of the Health & Social Care Act*, Nicholas Timmins.

6. 'NHS reforms our worst mistake, Tories admit', *The Times* 13/10/14.

Chapter 9

1. 'Wards in a fifth of NHS hospitals face the axe', *Telegraph* 5/10/12.

2. 'The strike is a symptom of an NHS in intensive care', *The Guardian* 13/10/14.

3. 'NHS trusts are enmeshed in private provision - as buyers and suppliers', *The Guardian* 18/12/12.

4. 'Integration? The opposite is true in Jeremy Hunt's NHS', *The Guardian* 11/10/12.

5. GPs put the squeeze on access to hospital care – British Medical Journal 10/7/2013 2013;347:f4432.

6. 'Devon - the canary in the NHS coalmine?', OpenDemocracy 4/12/14.

7. '£207m debt at PFI-saddled hospital trust "should be written off"', *Telegraph* 29/10/12.

8. 'Private Finance Initiative: hospitals will bring taxpayers 60 years of pain', *Telegraph* 24/1/11.

9. Lewisham Hospital: Appeal Court overrules Jeremy Hunt, *BBC News* 29/10/13.

10. Planning for closure: the role of special administrators in reducing NHS hospital services in England – British Medical Journal 13/12/132013;347:f7322 Allyson Pollock, David Price et al.

11. 'PFI hospital crisis: 20 more NHS trusts "at risk"', *Telegraph* 26/6/12.

12. Shaping a Healthier Future Pre-consultation Business Case, Appendix C, p.15.

13. NHAP condemns massive cuts in West London Hospitals, National Health Action Party statement 21/2/13.

14. 'Royal baby NHS trust to slash NHS beds and boost private income', *Evening Standard* 12/8/14.

15. 'Health boss pulls out of £120,000 taxpayer-funded "study tour"', *Evening Standard* 28/11/14.
16. 'The list of 66 A&E and maternity units being hit by cuts', *Telegraph* 26/10/14.
17. 'Lewisham is just the start of hospital protests to come', *The Guardian* 25/1/13.
18. 'NHS strike: Staff begin biggest strike in 30 years over 1% pay row', *The Independent* 13/10/14.
19. 'Hospitals and fire services to be run "outside the public sector"', *Telegraph* 14/12/14.
20. Mutual ownership: privatisation under a different name? British Medical Journal 21/8/14 2014;349:g5150 by Martin McKee.

Chapter 10

1. 'Patients with long term conditions can hold own budgets from 2015', *British Medical Journal News* 19/7/14.
2. 'More hospitals could be privately operated in NHS shakeup, says review', *The Guardian* 5/12/14.
3. 'Revealed: All new GP contracts will be thrown open to private providers', *Pulse Magazine* 18/8/14.
4. 'The real force behind the NHS Act - the EU/US trade agreement', Linda Kaucher, Open Democracy 19/2/13.
5. 'This transatlantic trade deal is a full-frontal assault on democracy', George Monbiot, *The Guardian* 4/11/13.
6. Trade secrets: will an EU-US treaty enable US big business to gain a foothold? – British Medical Journal 5/6/13 2013;346:f3574.
7. 'The NHS will fail us so long as we look on it as a market', *The Guardian* 8/8/13.
8. 'Scotland's prescription for health: ditch the PFI', *The Guardian* 22/1/14.
9. 'Will MPs vote to right some of the NHS wrongs?', *The Guardian* 18/11/13.

Contemporary culture has eliminated both the concept of the public and the figure of the intellectual. Former public spaces – both physical and cultural – are now either derelict or colonized by advertising. A cretinous anti-intellectualism presides, cheerled by expensively educated hacks in the pay of multinational corporations who reassure their bored readers that there is no need to rouse themselves from their interpassive stupor. The informal censorship internalized and propagated by the cultural workers of late capitalism generates a banal conformity that the propaganda chiefs of Stalinism could only ever have dreamt of imposing. Zer0 Books knows that another kind of discourse – intellectual without being academic, popular without being populist – is not only possible: it is already flourishing, in the regions beyond the striplit malls of so-called mass media and the neurotically bureaucratic halls of the academy. Zer0 is committed to the idea of publishing as a making public of the intellectual. It is convinced that in the unthinking, blandly consensual culture in which we live, critical and engaged theoretical reflection is more important than ever before.

ZERO BOOKS

If this book has helped you to clarify an idea, solve a problem or extend your knowledge, you may like to read more titles from Zero Books. Recent bestsellers are:

Capitalist Realism Is there no alternative?
Mark Fisher
An analysis of the ways in which capitalism has presented itself as the only realistic political-economic system.
Paperback: November 27, 2009 978-1-84694-317-1 $14.95 £7.99.
eBook: July 1, 2012 978-1-78099-734-6 $9.99 £6.99.

The Wandering Who? A study of Jewish identity politics
Gilad Atzmon
An explosive unique crucial book tackling the issues of Jewish Identity Politics and ideology and their global influence.
Paperback: September 30, 2011 978-1-84694-875-6 $14.95 £8.99.
eBook: September 30, 2011 978-1-84694-876-3 $9.99 £6.99.

Clampdown Pop-cultural wars on class and gender
Rhian E. Jones
Class and gender in Britpop and after, and why 'chav' is a feminist issue.
Paperback: March 29, 2013 978-1-78099-708-7 $14.95 £9.99.
eBook: March 29, 2013 978-1-78099-707-0 $7.99 £4.99.

The Quadruple Object
Graham Harman
Uses a pack of playing cards to present Harman's metaphysical system of fourfold objects, including human access, Heidegger's indirect causation, panpsychism and ontography.
Paperback: July 29, 2011 978-1-84694-700-1 $16.95 £9.99.

Weird Realism Lovecraft and Philosophy
Graham Harman
As Hölderlin was to Martin Heidegger and Mallarmé to Jacques
Derrida, so is H.P. Lovecraft to the Speculative Realist philoso-
phers.
Paperback: September 28, 2012 978-1-78099-252-5 $24.95 £14.99.
eBook: September 28, 2012 978-1-78099-907-4 $9.99 £6.99.

Sweetening the Pill or How We Got Hooked on Hormonal Birth
Control
Holly Grigg-Spall
Is it really true? Has contraception liberated or oppressed
women?
Paperback: September 27, 2013 978-1-78099-607-3 $22.95 £12.99.
eBook: September 27, 2013 978-1-78099-608-0 $9.99 £6.99.

Why Are We The Good Guys? Reclaiming Your Mind From The
Delusions Of Propaganda
David Cromwell
A provocative challenge to the standard ideology that Western
power is a benevolent force in the world.
Paperback: September 28, 2012 978-1-78099-365-2 $26.95 £15.99.
eBook: September 28, 2012 978-1-78099-366-9 $9.99 £6.99.

The Truth about Art Reclaiming quality
Patrick Doorly
The book traces the multiple meanings of art to their various
sources, and equips the reader to choose between them.
Paperback: August 30, 2013 978-1-78099-841-1 $32.95 £19.99.

Bells and Whistles More Speculative Realism
Graham Harman
In this diverse collection of sixteen essays, lectures, and inter-
views Graham Harman lucidly explains the principles of

Speculative Realism, including his own object-oriented philosophy.
Paperback: November 29, 2013 978-1-78279-038-9 $26.95 £15.99.
eBook: November 29, 2013 978-1-78279-037-2 $9.99 £6.99.

Towards Speculative Realism: Essays and Lectures Essays and Lectures
Graham Harman
These writings chart Harman's rise from Chicago sportswriter to co founder of one of Europe's most promising philosophical movements: Speculative Realism.
Paperback: November 26, 2010 978-1-84694-394-2 $16.95 £9.99.
eBook: January 1, 1970 978-1-84694-603-5 $9.99 £6.99.

Meat Market Female flesh under capitalism
Laurie Penny
A feminist dissection of women's bodies as the fleshy fulcrum of capitalist cannibalism, whereby women are both consumers and consumed.
Paperback: April 29, 2011 978-1-84694-521-2 $12.95 £6.99.
eBook: May 21, 2012 978-1-84694-782-7 $9.99 £6.99.

Translating Anarchy The Anarchism of Occupy Wall Street
Mark Bray
An insider's account of the anarchists who ignited Occupy Wall Street.
Paperback: September 27, 2013 978-1-78279-126-3 $26.95 £15.99.
eBook: September 27, 2013 978-1-78279-125-6 $6.99 £4.99.

One Dimensional Woman
Nina Power
Exposes the dark heart of contemporary cultural life by examining pornography, consumer capitalism and the ideology of women's work.

Paperback: November 27, 2009 978-1-84694-241-9 $14.95 £7.99.
eBook: July 1, 2012 978-1-78099-737-7 $9.99 £6.99.

Dead Man Working
Carl Cederstrom, Peter Fleming
An analysis of the dead man working and the way in which
capital is now colonizing life itself.
Paperback: May 25, 2012 978-1-78099-156-6 $14.95 £9.99.
eBook: June 27, 2012 978-1-78099-157-3 $9.99 £6.99.

Unpatriotic History of the Second World War
James Heartfield
The Second World War was not the Good War of legend. James
Heartfield explains that both Allies and Axis powers fought for
the same goals - territory, markets and natural resources.
Paperback: September 28, 2012 978-1-78099-378-2 $42.95 £23.99.
eBook: September 28, 2012 978-1-78099-379-9 $9.99 £6.99.

Find more titles at www.zero-books.net